Risk Assessment and Risk Communication Strategies in Bioterrorism Preparedness

T0137948

NATO Security through Science Series

This Series presents the results of scientific meetings supported under the NATO Programme for Security through Science (STS).

Meetings supported by the NATO STS Programme are in security-related priority areas of Defence Against Terrorism or Countering Other Threats to Security. The types of meeting supported are generally "Advanced Study Institutes" and "Advanced Research Workshops". The NATO STS Series collects together the results of these meetings. The meetings are co-organized by scientists from NATO countries and scientists from NATO's "Partner" or "Mediterranean Dialogue" countries. The observations and recommendations made at the meetings, as well as the contents of the volumes in the Series, reflect those of participants and contributors only; they should not necessarily be regarded as reflecting NATO views or policy.

Advanced Study Institutes (ASI) are high-level tutorial courses to convey the latest developments in a subject to an advanced-level audience

Advanced Research Workshops (ARW) are expert meetings where an intense but informal exchange of views at the frontiers of a subject aims at identifying directions for future action

Following a transformation of the programme in 2004 the Series has been re-named and re-organised. Recent volumes on topics not related to security, which result from meetings supported under the programme earlier, may be found in the NATO Science Series.

The Series is published by IOS Press, Amsterdam, and Springer, Dordrecht, in conjunction with the NATO Public Diplomacy Division.

Sub-Series

A. Chemistry and Biology	Springer
B. Physics and Biophysics	Springer
C. Environmental Security	Springer
D. Information and Communication Security	IOS Press
E. Human and Societal Dynamics	IOS Press

http://www.nato.int/science
http://www.springer.com
http://www.iospress.nl

Series A: Chemistry and Biology

Risk Assessment and Risk Communication Strategies in Bioterrorism Preparedness

edited by

Manfred S. Green
Faculty of Medicine, Tel Aviv University,
Israel

Jonathan Zenilman
Johns Hopkins Bloomberg School of Public Health, Baltimore, MD,
U.S.A.

Dani Cohen
Faculty of Medicine, Tel Aviv University,
Israel

Itay Wiser
Faculty of Medicine, Tel Aviv University,
Israel

and

Ran D. Balicer
Ben-Gurion University of the Negev, Beer-Sheva,
Israel

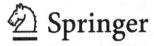 Springer

Published in cooperation with NATO Public Diplomacy Division

Proceedings of the NATO Advanced Research Workshop on
Risk Assessment and Risk Communication in Bioterrorism
Ein-Gedi, Israel
June, 2005

A C.I.P. Catalogue record for this book is available from the Library of Congress.

ISBN 978-1-4020-5806-6 (HB)
ISBN 978-1-4020-5808-0 (eBook)

Published by Springer,
P.O. Box 17, 3300 AA Dordrecht, The Netherlands.

www.springer.com

Printed on acid-free paper

CONTENTS

Preface ix

Part I   RISK ASSESSMENT 1

1. INTRODUCTION TO BIOTERRORISM RISK
   ASSESSMENT 3
   Ran D. Balicer and Itay Wiser

2. SOME PUBLIC HEALTH PERSPECTIVES
   ON QUANTITATIVE RISK ASSESSMENTS
   FOR BIOTERRORISM 19
   Steve Leach

3. SITUATIONAL AWARENESS IN A BIOTERROR ATTACK
   VIA PROBABILITY MODELING 31
   Edward H. Kaplan and Johan Walden

4. THE BIOTERRORISM THREAT 45
   Yair Sharan

5. CHANGE OF MIND-SET FOLLOWING 9/11: THE FEW THAT
   ARE ALREADY WILLING TO RESORT TO WEAPONS
   OF MASS DESTRUCTION 55
   Yoram Schweitzer

6. ANTIMICROBIAL PROPHYLAXIS AND PROVIDING
   SUBACUTE CARE IN THE CONTEXT
   OF A BIOTERRORISM EVENT: LESSONS LEARNED
   FROM 2001 67
   Jonathan Zenilman

7. DETECTING AND RESPONDING TO BIOTERRORISM 77
   Janet Martha Blatny

8. SPECIES-NEUTRAL DISEASE SURVEILLANCE:
   A FOUNDATION OF RISK ASSESSMENT
   AND COMMUNICATION 93
   David R. Franz

Part II   RISK COMMUNICATION 101

9. **INTRODUCTION TO BIOTERRORISM RISK COMMUNICATION** 103
   Itay Wiser and Ran D. Balicer

10. **RISK COMMUNICATION TO HEALTH-CARE WORKERS AS A RISK REDUCTION MEASURE IN BIOTERRORISM** 117
    Yoav Yehezkelli, Yoram Amsalem, and Adi Aran

11. **ANTHRAX-EURONET AND BEYOND – CHALLENGES OF SCIENTIFIC RESEARCH ON HIGH RISK AGENTS** 123
    Amanda J. Ozin and Stephen H.E. Kaufmann

12. **RISK COMMUNICATION AND PUBLIC BEHAVIOR IN EMERGENCIES** 131
    Yair Amikam

13. **PREVENTION STRATEGIES AND PROMOTING PSYCHOLOGICAL RESILIENCE TO BIOTERRORISM THROUGH COMMUNICATION** 135
    Anne Speckhard

14. **RISK COMMUNICATION AND THE COMMUNITY RESPONSE TO A BIOTERRORIST ATTACK: THE ROLE OF AN INTERNET-BASED EARLY WARNING SYSTEM A.K.A. "THE INFORMAL SECTOR"** 163
    Marjorie Pollack

15. **INFORMATION SYSTEMS FOR RISK COMMUNICATION RELATED TO BIOTERRORISM** 177
    Manfred S. Green and Zalamn Kaufman

Part III   FOCUS ON SMALLPOX 193

16. **RISK ASSESSMENT IN SMALLPOX BIOTERRORIST AGGRESSION** 195
    Marian Negut

17. **RENEWAL OF IMMUNOLOGICAL MEMORY TO SMALLPOX: USE OF NEW TOOLS YIELDS OLD RESULTS** 205
    Jonathan Boxman, Itay Wiser, and Nadav Orr

18. PREPARING FOR A SMALLPOX BIOTERRORIST
ATTACK: PULSE VACCINATION
AS AN OPTIMAL STRATEGY 219
Zvia Agur, Karen Marron, Hanita Shai, and Yehuda L. Danon

ADDITIONAL ABSTRACTS 231

19. A PRIORI VERSUS A POSTERIORI RISK ASSESSMENT
FOR BIOTERROR ATTACK 233
Eli Stern

20. IMPACT OF THE PROLIFERATION OF WEAPONS
OF MASS DESTRUCTION ON THE STABILITY
IN THE MIDDLE EAST 235
M.K. Shiyyab

21. THE ROLE OF RISK ASSESSMENT IN PREPARING
THE HEALTH-CARE SYSTEM FOR BIOTERRORISM
AND NATURAL EPIDEMICS 237
Meir Oren

22. SUSCEPTIBILITY OF *B. ANTHRACIS* TO VARIOUS
ANTIBACTERIAL AGENTS AND THEIR TIME-KILL
ACTIVITY 239
Abed Athamna and Ethan Rubinstein

23. NATURAL OR INTENTIONAL FOOD CONTAMINATION?
HOW CAN WE KNOW? 241
Daniel Cohen

24. BIOTERRORISM EMERGENCY RESPONSE:
CURRENT CONCEPTS AND CONTROVERSIES 243
Eric. K. Noji

25. PREPAREDNESS AND RESPONSE FOR BIOTERRORISM
INVOLVING THE FOOD SUPPLY 245
Jeremy Sobel

26. RISK COMMUNICATION AND PSYCHOLOGICAL
IMPACT: TECHNOLOGICAL AND OPERATIONAL
METHODS OF MITIGATION 247
Michael J. Hopmeier

PREFACE

Biological weapons have been used since ancient history, mostly by armies in the field of battle, or in siege. Following the rapid development of biological weapons in the 20th century, bioterrorism became a new reality. In recent years, several incidents have occurred; perhaps the most dramatic was that of the anthrax envelopes in the United States in 2001. Bioterrorism can cause damage both directly and indirectly. The first and obvious damage is illness and death caused by the agent used. However, this may be a relatively minor part of the overall damage. Public anxiety and fear resulting from a bioterrorist event can have a devastating effect on the society. In dealing with bioterrorism, comprehensive risk assessment is necessary to ensure that the resources needed to deal with the incident are available. In addition, an effective risk communication plan must be developed in advance.

Risk assessment is essential to determine and prioritize potential future vulnerabilities based on solid facts. Careful analysis will help quantify the impact of possible countermeasures on the existing risks. The process of risk assessment includes creating possible scenarios of bioterrorism using present knowledge of the organisms that may be used, the preferred targets, methods of spread, etc. This is followed by an assessment of the likelihood of different scenarios, based on both the motivation of different terrorist groups and their capabilities in terms of laboratory knowledge, pathogens held, and distribution abilities. In the risk assessment, consequences of possible scenarios can be estimated using methods of exposure assessment, data on natural epidemics, and from laboratory studies. The possible countermeasures against a bioterrorist event can be examined in the risk assessment models, and chosen accordingly.

Since the goal of bioterrorism is to spread fear and panic among the public, effective risk communication is essential. Risk communication is a field that analyses and suggests alternative ways to communicate with the public in times of crisis and public risk. Good risk communication practices that are applied early and continually can help mitigate the panic and direct the public toward constructive steps thus helping them to deal with the consequences of a bioterrorist incident.

In light of the risks presented by the increasing threat of bioterrorism, we proposed that a North Atlantic Treaty Organization (NATO) Advanced Research Workshop on the subject of "The role of risk assessment and risk communication in bioterrorism" be held in Israel. The aim of the workshop was to generate discussion among leading experts in the field of risk assessment, risk communication, and bioterrorism in order to form new strategies and improve present strategies to deal with a bioterrorist threat. We hoped to create an interdisciplinary, multinational group to further discuss and develop risk assessment and communication policy, and applications. The workshop was held in the city of Eilat, situated between Jordan in the east and Egypt in the west.

In the course of three days, current knowledge and future trends concerning risk management in bioterrorism were presented. The heart of the workshop was the discussion groups that took place at the end of each session. The final day of the workshop was dedicated to preparing a summary document containing the main points discussed and a plan for future research and development of risk management strategies. This book contains the papers that resulted from the workshop and it should be an invaluable reference for all involved in countering bioterrorism.

Manfred S Green and Jonathan Zenilman
Co-directors of the Workshop

Part I

RISK ASSESSMENT

INTRODUCTION TO BIOTERRORISM RISK ASSESSMENT

Ran D. Balicer[1] and Itay Wiser[2]
[1] *Ran D. Balicer, MD, MPH*
Epidemiology Department, Faculty of Health Sciences, Ben-Gurion
University of the Negav, Beer-Sheva, Israel
[2] *Itay Wiser: MD. Department of Epidemiology and Preventive*
Medicine, School of Public Health, Sackler Faculty of Medicine,
Tel Aviv University

1.   Pre-event

1.1.   WHY HAS BIOTERRORISM NOT BEEN USED SO FAR TO PROMOTE POLITICAL AGENDAS/VIEWS?

A quantitative risk assessment depends on there being some reliable data available to the analyst. A quantitative bioterrorism risk assessment would need data or well-informed judgments on the intent of terrorist groups or individuals, their technical capabilities, the attributes of pathogens or toxins that might be used in a biological attack, target characteristics, and the occurrence (frequency) of various attack scenarios. While data regarding target and bioagent characteristics are available, to a lesser or greater extent, data on bioterrorist intent and the frequency of different types of attacks are just about nonexistent.

This data gap apparently stems from the rarity of bioterrorist events and the need to better understand the motives of the terrorists themselves. To illustrate, a search of the Center for Nonproliferation Studies (CNS) weapons of mass destruction (WMD) terrorism database, which is the largest unclassified one of its kind, revealed that out of 383 incidents in which biological, chemical, nuclear, or radiological agents were used by criminals or terrorists during 1900–2001, only 77 biological "events" (i.e., episodes involving the deliberate use of a biological agent to harm people) were perpetrated. Of these, just four post-1945 events generated more than 10 casualties [1].

The successful implementation of a bioterrorism act would require the achievement of several critical steps by the terrorist: acquiring precursor virulent biological seed cultures, growing biological agents in culture,

M.S. Green et al. (eds.), Risk Assessment and Risk Communication Strategies in Bioterrorism
Preparedness, 3–17.
© 2007 *Springer.*

process the agents into a form that can be effectively disseminated, improvise an agent delivery device, and carry out the dissemination effectively to cause mass casualties [2]. Even when the appropriate motivation for such an attack exists, an actual effective attack can only be carried out once each of these obstacles has been overcome. Obtaining the appropriate microorganism to initiate an event requires access, as well as knowledge. Restrictions in distribution of potential bioterrorist agents have reduced such accessibility. In addition, the most appropriate strain must be selected. It is speculated that one reason for the lack of success at disseminating anthrax by the cult Aum Shinrikio was the inadvertent selection of a nonpathogenic strain of *Bacillus anthracis* [2].

Reviewing small portions of the peer-reviewed literature of the past several years, authors have found numerous articles that might be considered useful to would-be bioweaponeers. Published advances in the life sciences that arguably have dual-use applications can be found in many diverse fields, including directed evolution; studies of the mechanisms of virulence in viruses and bacteria including human, animal, and plant pathogens; gene therapy technology; aerosol technology; bio-manufacturing; and so on. Efforts are made to limit the available data on bioterrorism agents in the literature, which may be used by terrorists in their attempts to produce agents of bioterrorism [3]. Yet some authors claim restrictions are already too restrictive, and may have adverse outcomes [4]. Efforts to monitor comprehensively all bioscience research that has potentially destructive applications would subsume huge swaths of science, gravely tax civilian research resources, and could discourage scientists from pursuing advances in fields important to medicine and agriculture, fields we urgently need to advance in order to address the grave vulnerabilities currently imposed by bioweapons [3].

Some authors further believe we grossly overestimate the importance of the threat of bioterrorism. They point out that we must recognize a conflict of interest exists, and that it is an important, though often neglected, element in public health priority setting. They compare these to the conflicts of interest in prevention of the health consequences of tobacco use or of environmental pollution, such as the desire for profit through the provision of equipment, supplies, or consultation, for prestige through the public, visible role in prevention or preparedness, and for power though partici-pation in planning and execution of prevention or preparedness programs. The enormous federal investment in bioterrorism preparedness in the United States has generated enormous profit, prestige, and power to those who engage it [5].

1.1.1. Do we really believe "they" have the capabilities to execute an attack using anthrax, smallpox?

Most authors believe the risk of a smallpox attack is fairly low. The known supplies of variola virus are limited, rogue states with the virus would probably fear "boomerang" effects or devastating retaliation, and terrorists are unlikely to be capable of successfully handling a lethal mammalian virus [6].

Examining the 2001 anthrax events in hindsight, it appears that neither the targets of attack, nor the person or group responsible for attacks, could have been predetermined by any known prediction methodology. When scientific knowledge about probabilities is absent, thinking about possible outcomes takes on a particular significance [1,7].

One suggested partial remedy for such lack of data regarding the intent and ability of the perpetrators to perform an act of bioterrorism, can therefore be vulnerability analysis. A vulnerability analysis seeks to identify a valuable asset (i.e., a target) at risk of a bioterrorist attack and to concept-ualize various ways in which it is vulnerable to such an attack (i.e., various attack scenarios). Accordingly, what might have been predicted in the case of anthrax was that the US mail system could not only be used as a means to deliver anthrax, but also that a letter containing anthrax spores could spread spores among mail workers and to other recipients of mail besides the intended victims, through transfer of spores from the original letter to other pieces of mail. Zilinskas and colleagues further detail these concepts in their summary of a workshop on Bioterrorism Threat Assessment and Risk Management [1].

1.2. CAN THEY REALLY SPREAD THESE AGENTS EFFECTIVELY?

Most biological agents (especially type A) are most effectively used as an aerosol. Effective delivery of an aerosolized agent requires that the particle size be 1–10 μm to be able to reach the terminal bronchioles and alveoli. Successful aerosol dispersion of a biological agent is also inherently dependent on the environmental and meteorological conditions.

Models calculating the number of casualties inflicted by an aerosol attack have ranged in hundreds of thousands to the millions. Theoretically an air-craft dispersing 100 kg of anthrax over a 300 km^2 area could cause three million deaths in a population density of 10,000 people per km. Aerosolized botulinum toxin has been estimated to decay at between 1% and 4% per min, depending on the ambient temperature. At a decay rate of 1% per min, substantial inactivation ($\geq$13 logs) of toxin occurs by 2 days after aerosoliza-tion. In the case of plague, the major shortcoming is that it is inactivated by sunlight. On the other hand, unlike anthrax and botulinum toxin, it is capable of being transmitted from person to person. However, as evidenced by the recent anthrax letters of 2001, aerosolization of an agent via a plane or machine may not be needed to strike fear and uncertainty among the public [8].

Dissemination of a category A biological agent through the contamination of food and water is considered less likely as most category A agents are not effectively transmitted via food and water. Although category B agents can be transmitted by these routes, they usually cause only short-term vomiting and diarrhea, with a relatively quick recovery. Present public water treatment methods, as well as the boiling of water and cooking of food, are highly effective in neutralizing many biological agents. Contaminating a water or food supply effectively would require large amounts of toxin and bacteria to overcome any dilution factor. However, a recent study warns of the United States' vulnerability to such an attack based on very centralized food processing and distribution methods over large areas. Likely agents are botulinum toxin, *Salmonella*, *Shigella*, *Escherichia coli*, and *Vibrio cholerae*. The proposed use of botulinum toxin to contaminate a public water source is of questionable efficacy as the amount of botulinum toxin needed to effectively negate any dilution factor would be enormous, as well as the fact that it is naturally deactivated in fresh water within 3–6 days and within 20 min of standard water treatment. In terms of contamination of a food supply, it should be noted that the toxin is inactivated by heating food to 85°C [8].

Infection via contact of intact skin with any of the agents is unlikely to result in casualties. However, if the skin integrity is compromised, the potential for disease exists. The recent anthrax letters resulted in 11 cases of cutaneous anthrax causing significant disruption and fear in postal services and mail handlers. Current studies suggest that thorough washing with soap and water is sufficient to overcome even this threat. Currently, with the exception of anthrax, none of the category A agents have environmental stability after release, especially outdoors [8].

Table 1 summarizes the dissemination techniques employed so far in bioterrorism events [2].

TABLE 1. Dissemination techniques employed [7]

Type	Terrorist	Criminal	Other/uncertain	Total incidents
Aerosol dissemination	2	0	0	2
Direct injection/topical application	6	10	0	16
Contaminated food	1	20	1	22
Contaminated water	4	0	2	6
Insect/natural vectors	0	1	1	2
None	10	13	79	102
Unknown	5	10	2	17
Total cases	28	54	85	

1.3. REGARDING SMALLPOX: WHAT NEW EVIDENCE WOULD JUSTIFY, ACCORDING TO CURRENTLY ACCEPTED MODELS AND ESTIMATES, PRE-EVENT VACCINATION OF THE WHOLE POPULATION OR SPECIFIC SUBPOPULATIONS?

The most important risks associated with pre-event smallpox vaccination program are the adverse events associated with significant morbidity and those for which there are no screening criteria to reduce risk. On the basis of these criteria, post-vaccinial encephalitis and the newly appreciated cardiac complications, especially myopericarditis, are of greatest concern [6].

The risk–benefit ratio associated with pre-event smallpox vaccination program would depend on several factors, including mainly the probability for an event and the potential impact of the event, which in turn is largely determined by the site attacked and means of dispersion. One stochastic model, for example, has shown pre-event vaccination of health-care workers proves lifesaving if the probability of a building attack exceeded 0.22 or if the probability of a high-impact airport attack exceeded 0.002. However, from a national policy standpoint, at the "breakeven" thresholds, the policy implications of vaccination are not equivalent to the policy implications of forgoing vaccination. Forgoing prior vaccination means risking higher losses in an attack for a high probability (for instance 0.78) that there will be no attack and no deaths. In contrast, instituting prior vaccination ensures that losses will be lower, should an attack occur, but requires acceptance of the certainty of many vaccine-related deaths and considerable morbidity [9].

The authors of the above-cited model endorsed in their conclusions "a policy of vaccinating all eligible health care workers and first responders before an attack." They assumed that these workers would accept the "risk of personal harm for the public good" and would volunteer to get vaccinated, which has turned out not to be the case. If civilian medical care and public health workers were reluctant to get vaccinated in the face of a much smaller risk of post-vaccinial encephalitis, will they be less reluctant and volunteer in the face of an additionally recognized myopericarditis risk of 1 in 1,800? [6].

TABLE 2. Direct risks and benefits of pre-event smallpox vaccination before and after a smallpox outbreak [6]

Perspective	Risks realized before an outbreak	Benefits realized before an outbreak	Benefits realized after an outbreak
Individual			
Individual (vaccinees)	Severe adverse reactions, including death[a] Employment risks[a] Financial risks[a]	Psychological benefits ("peace of mind," sense of contributing to public good)	Protection against smallpox, including death
Contact (e.g., patient)	Contact vaccinia[b]	None	Protection against smallpox from vaccinated contact
Population			
Public health and medical sectors	Contact vaccinia (low risk)[b]	Increased preparedness, practice, and readiness from administering the vaccine and running vaccination clinics Increased clinical knowledge from management of adverse events Increased availability of vaccinia immune globulin Increase in scientific knowledge from studying vaccinees	Prevaccinated vaccinators[d] More efficient and timely mass vaccination campaign[d] Prevaccinated medical care teams to care for smallpox patients[d] Prevaccinated public health response teams (investigation, contact tracing, vaccination)[d] Better clinical management of adverse reactions from mass vaccination Better availability of vaccinia immune globulin
General public	Contact vaccinia (very low risk)[b] Possible decreased trust in health authorities[c]	Increase in scientific knowledge from studying vaccinees Possible increased trust in health authorities[c] Deterrent to terrorists	All benefits described previously Some herd immunity Increased trust in health authorities

[a] The informed consent process emphasizes the disclosure of the individual health, employment, and financial risks to the vaccinee.

[b] The risk of contact vaccinia will increase as vaccination becomes more widespread among vaccinees not well trained in infection control practices.

[c] The level of trust or mistrust of health authorities will depend on several factors, including how honestly and effectively health officials communicate the risks, benefits, and trade-offs from the different stakeholder perspectives summarized in this table.

[d] The post-outbreak response benefits from pre-event vaccination could be small if pre-event planning, preparedness, and readiness are not optimal. For example, vaccinated but untrained public health response workers would still need to be trained, potentially delaying an effective response. Additionally, efficient post-outbreak mass and ring vaccination could mitigate the risks from lack of pre-event vaccination.

2.   Once an Outbreak Occurs

2.1.   CAN WE PREDICT THE DISSEMINATION PATTERNS AND MAGNITUDE OF THE OUTBREAK AT ITS FIRST STAGES? WHAT DATA SHOULD WE QUICKLY COLLECT TO FACILITATE SUCH EMERGENCY MODELING EFFORTS?

During public health emergencies, such as bioterrorist attacks and disease epidemics, computerized information systems for data management, analysis, and communication may be needed within hours of beginning the investigation. Available sources of data and output requirements of the system may be changed frequently during the course of the investigation. Integrating data from a variety of sources may require entering or importing data from a variety of digital and paper formats. Spatial representation of data is particularly valuable for assessing environmental exposure [10].

One study suggests an approach, which attempts to reduce the complexity of the problem space by finding clusters of similar threats. Because our focus is the design of information systems, the clustering of threats is based on similarities in the functional requirements that each threat imposes on a detection system – threats with similar functional requirements for detection are grouped together. The goal of this approach is to develop a parsimonious and tractable characterization of the problem space for the purpose of surveillance system design, one that will facilitate both design of systems and the associated research in public health surveillance that supports system design. The consequence is that a designer feels confident that as long as clear specifications for detection of one threat in a category are met, the resulting system can detect any threat from the category. The potential advantages of such parsimonious characterization are: (1) focusing more attention on a smaller, but more comprehensive set of threats, (2) identifying equivalent threats that may be more amenable to study because of availability of data, and (3) improving tractability of analysis without, ideally, loss of generality [11].

But even when we attempt to focus at one disease, major uncertainties hinder our ability to reach valid and robust conclusions. In the smallpox case, it is unclear how much residual immunity remains today as a result of past vaccination programs; those vaccinated 25–30 years ago are unlikely to possess complete immunity and a significant proportion may develop less severe forms of the disease, potentially changing the dynamics of transmission. Allowing for past immunity levels is therefore critical when estimating R_0 from historical data. Historically, most infections occurred in caregivers to symptomatic individuals, whether in households or hospitals

[3]. It is unclear how 30 years of changes in household sizes, working patterns, and mobility would affect transmission patterns today. Incorporating detailed data on demographics and human mobility into spatially explicit models offers one method by which such extrapolation can be made more reliable, but the scale of changes mean that much uncertainty will inevitably remain. With such uncertainty, it is critical that risk assessment studies use modern statistical methods to obtain the best possible parameter estimates from historical data, while allowing for changes in the last 30 years. However, historical data are less relevant for some key parameters – such as the likely scale of a bioterrorist attack, how rapidly the disease would be recognized, and the ability of public health authorities to respond. Furthermore, it is unclear how population behavior would change in the face of an epidemic. Before recognition of the outbreak, would individuals in the latter stages of prodrome have more or fewer contacts, compared with their historical counterparts? Once smallpox is identified, will people voluntarily restrict their movements, or attempt to flee urban centers? These factors need to be explored with robust analysis of the sensitivity of model results and predicted optimal controls to parameter assumptions [12].

A variety of methods exist for controlling the spread of smallpox, ranging from different vaccination strategies to movement/contact restrictions placed on infectious cases and their contacts. Thus a key aspect of policy-orientated epidemic modeling is to assess both the adequacy of current policy and how it might further be optimized. Optimality is principally the minimization of mortality and morbidity, so it is critical that models accurately incorporate expected adverse event rates from vaccination. However, the severe acute respiratory syndrome (SARS) virus has shown that the economic costs of an epidemic can be out of all proportion to the numbers infected, indicating that minimizing the duration of a smallpox outbreak might also be a critical priority when formulating control strategy [12].

2.2.   CAN WE PREDICT THE EFFECT OF INTERVENTIONS DURING AN EVENT? CAN WE TRUST MODELS THAT SUGGEST LIMITED RESPONSE (I.E., TARGETED RATHER THAN MASS VACCINATION FOR SMALLPOX) SHOULD BE SUFFICIENT?

In every scenario, policymakers must choose between several intervention options for controlling the emerging epidemic. Table 3 by Ferguson et al. summarizes the main options for controlling a smallpox attack [12].

TABLE 3. Policy options for controlling smallpox attack [12]

Policy	Benefits	Drawbacks
Quarantine/isolation Quarantine and isolation of suspect and confirmed cases	If isolation facilities are adequate, it is highly effective at reducing transmission from known cases	Isolation facilities necessary, or compliance with voluntary policy. Compulsory policies necessarily coercive. Requires rapid detection of cases.
Movement restrictions For example, quarantine of neighborhoods or closure of schools, airports, or other transport systems	Potentially useful in containing a small outbreak where community transmission is occurring. Used recently to control SARS spread in Hong Kong and Singapore	Vaccination certificates issued in the past to prevent potential spread but difficult to assess effectiveness. Costly and difficult to police, compromised by any illegal movements. Coercive
"Ring" vaccination Contacts of suspect smallpox cases are traced and vaccinated when found. Can be coupled with policy of isolation of identified contacts	Minimizes use of vaccine, and hence morbidity and mortality caused by adverse reactions to vaccination	Contacts need to be found at an early stage of incubation for vaccine to be effective. Tracing needs to be highly effective to severely limit transmission
Targeted vaccination For example, vaccination of whole population in affected neighborhood or city	Highly effective during eradication campaign at containing transmission localized to a single geographic area or subpopulation. Reduced vaccine-related mortality. Not dependent on contact tracing	Effective when background levels of herd immunity high, but few systematic data on effectiveness in other contexts. Less sparing of vaccine use than ring vaccination. Risk of disease spreading beyond targeted area
Mass vaccination Vaccination of whole population of a country experiencing or threatened by an outbreak.	Effective at stopping widespread dissemination of the virus across large areas and protecting individuals from infection. Not dependent on contact tracing	Large numbers need to be vaccinated quickly. Might generate unnecessary vaccine-related morbidity and mortality. If policy implemented rapidly, screening for risk factors for adverse reactions might be suboptimal
Prophylactic vaccination Vaccination before a smallpox release	Useful for protecting essential 'first responder' personnel. If used for entire population, very effective at stopping widespread dissemination of virus. Does not have to be implemented quickly. Not dependent on contact tracing	If used to protect an entire population on an ongoing basis, policy has high, long-term cost, and a large number of probably unnecessary vaccine-associated adverse events would be expected for as long as policy is followed

When attempting to choose the most appropriate of these response policies prior to an actual event, analyses highlight the importance of beliefs regarding the nature of a bioterrorist attack and response logistics, in addition to disease epidemiology. In the case of smallpox, several examples may be considered. Would an attack be small and controllable through traced vaccination or large enough to require mass vaccination? Would an attack be overt, in which case it could prove possible to respond immediately in a highly targeted fashion and obtain much better results or covert and detected only from symptomatic cases as assumed in this chapter? If traced vaccination was used in response to an attack, would tracing prove accurate and efficient (as documented for a highly unusual natural outbreak that occurred in a Nigerian town) or inaccurate (as suggested by a simulated large attack in a metropolitan area with population 10 million)? Could a rapid mass vaccination campaign be mounted soon enough after an attack occurs and with sufficiently high population coverage to avert most of the second-generation infections, but with care to avoid vaccine complications among those with contraindications? Having never faced a deliberate smallpox attack, there are no empiric answers to questions such as these. In particular, it is an *assumption* to pretend that parameters such as R_0 are known, even if estimated on the basis of past outbreaks, because such outbreaks could bear no resemblance to what could occur in a bioterrorist attack [13].

Several models have addressed the issue of choosing the optimal response policy for smallpox outbreak. Table 4 by Ferguson et al. summarizes several of these models, along with the author's views and comments for each of these models [12].

Similar dilemmas exist regarding an anthrax attack. One dilemma is how to rapidly identify such an attack, while preventing false alarms and unnecessary expenditures. The lack of sufficient experience with bioterrorism related pathogens, such as anthrax, might be a leading cause of delay in identifying bioterrorist event due to misdiagnosis. Using risk assessment methods, an effort is made to identify quickly and cost-effectively the first cases or exclude a bioterrorist event possibility. The main obstacle that stands in the experts' way is the insufficient existing data on which to rely on [14].

Another dilemma in the case of anthrax, live in evaluating the trade-off between the consequences of antibiotic use and the consequences of failure to treat anthrax poses a dilemma to the treating physician. One study suggests that during influenza season, rapid testing for influenza should be

TABLE 4. Summary of recent smallpox modeling studies [12]

Study	Key features	Comments
Meltzer, M. I., Damon, I., LeDuc, J. W. & Millar, J. D. Modeling potential responses to smallpox as a bioterrorist weapon. Emerg. Inf. Dis. 7, 959–969 (2001).	(1) Homogeneous mixing; (2) stochastic; (3) no social/ spatial structure; (4) $R_0 = 1.5–3$; (5) vaccination not directly modeled but in conjunction with quarantine is assumed to reduce R below 1; (6) no depletion of susceptibles; (7) 100 people initially infected	(1) Estimates required control effort by correlating vaccine doses used against number of cases in historical outbreaks; (2) number of doses is not related to the number of cases, but to the level of susceptibility (and R_0); (3) model substantially overestimates cases because depletion of susceptibles is not modeled;(4) controls assumed to reduce R to 0.99, that is, program effectiveness is model input
Kaplan, E. H., Craft, D. L. & Wein, L. M. Emergency response to a smallpox attack: The case for mass vaccination. Proc. Natl. Acad. Sci. USA 99, 10935–10940 (2002).	(1) Homogeneous mixing in large population (10 million); (2) deterministic; (3) no social/spatial structure; (4) $R_0 = 3$ for base case (range 1–20); (5) mass vaccination and ring vaccination compared; (6) considers public health logistical constraints; (7) only those "asymptomatic" (that is in prodrome) are infectious – those symptomatic (with rash) are assumed to be isolated; (8) number initially infected = 1–100,000	(1) R_0 assumed derived from historical estimates, but level of prodromal transmission assumed much greater than new best estimates derived from historical data[21]; (2) assumption that transmission occurs during the prodromal period biases results in favor of mass vaccination; (3) assumption of homogeneous mixing will also bias the results in favor of mass vaccination; (4) considers vaccine-related deaths only in contraindicated people, and not those in noncontraindicated individuals or other adverse events
Halloran, M. E., Longini, I. M., Nizam, A. & Yang. Y. Containing bioterrorist smallpox. Science 298, 1428–1432 (2002).	(1) Heterogeneous mixing (social structure included) in small population (2,000); (2) stochastic; (3) $R_0 = 3.2$; (4) mass vaccination and ring vaccination compared; (5) considers current residual herd immunity; (6) number initially infected = 1–10	(1) Large number of parameters assumed, particularly regarding mixing patterns, limited sensitivity analysis performed; (2) relatively large proportion (0.05–0.5%) of community initially infected; (3) model of small community of 2,000 individuals; (4) assumption that >75% of transmission occurs during prodrome biases results in favor of mass vaccination
Bozzette, S. A. et al. A model for a smallpox-vaccination policy. N. Engl. J. Med. 348, 416–425 (2003).	(1) Homogeneous mixing; (2) stochastic; (3) R(no control) = 15, 3.4 and 1.8 in hospital, mixed and community outbreaks respectively; ($R_0 \geq R$ (no control)); (4) compares mass vaccination, ring vaccination and prophylactic vaccination of healthcare workers; (5) considers vaccine-related adverse events; (6) number initially infected = 2–100,000	(1) Assumes the effect of the control policies on R, based on review and "judgment"; that is, effectiveness of policies is an input into the model rather than an output; the model therefore has little explanatory or predictive power; (2) large number of parameters assumed, limited sensitivity analysis performed; (3) assumes disease has no effect on the depletion of susceptibles; (4) assessment of threat of attack is subjective

performed in symptomatic patients, followed by empiric treatment for anthrax, pending blood culture results for those who test negative for influenza [15].

2.3. HOW DIFFERENT SHOULD INTENTIONALLY DISTRIBUTED SMALLPOX BE COMPARED TO NATURALLY OCCURRING SMALLPOX OUTBREAKS IN THE PAST?

If an attack occurs in the near future, it is unlikely that a genetically modified strain of variola would be used. However, if the strain is genetically modified to increase its virulence, possible consequences could be even more dramatic. Unfortunately, scientific advancements over the last two decades have made it possible to develop genetically altered strains of orthopoxviruses [16].

Genetic engineering of viruses has become a common practice. One major objective of genetic manipulation is to use engineered viral vectors for the delivery of genetic information with therapeutic intent or to modify viruses so as to alter the host's immune response. Changes in virulence and host range of modified viruses are generally hard to predict. However, when one studies the possibility of making variola virus more pathogenic, the research and development (R&D) work will most likely be focused on targets such as:

1. Shortening the incubation period of the disease by improving the attachment of the virus to a host cell and accelerating virus propagation in host cells
2. Reducing the infectious dose and increasing mortality by the suppression/subversion of innate and specific immune responses to the virus
3. Strengthening the severity, "adding" new syndromes of infection and increasing mortality by widening the number of potential sites of infection (e.g., brain and parenchymal organs).

These are just some of the possible targets of genetic engineering procedures. However, even if such work is underway in some countries, it is obvious that we would never obtain any "official" information on the work with variola virus to increase its virulence by inserting alien genes. At the same time, we need to know what and how this genetic engineering work could be performed in order to understand what protection we must develop against genetically engineered variola virus [16].

2.4. HOW SUSCEPTIBLE IS THE POPULATION TODAY TO SMALLPOX?

Routine smallpox vaccination program in Israel instituted in 1949, included vaccine administration to (i) infants aged 1 year, (ii) children (aged 9–10 years), (iii) military recruits (aged 18 years), and (iv) new immigrants. After the World Health Organization (WHO) declaration on the eradication of smallpox in 1979, routine smallpox vaccination in Israel was officially discontinued in July 1980. Army recruits continued to receive smallpox vaccination until July 1996. A first responder revaccination campaign began on September 2002 and as of May 2003, some 22,000 doses have been administered [17].

Data collected during the eradication campaign showed that neutralizing antibodies to smallpox are persistent and may be detected 20 years or more after vaccination [18]. More recent studies reported that after two revaccinations, the antibody levels to vaccinia persist and may provide a sufficient level of immunity for 30–75 years [19, 20]. Similar conclusions were drawn by Crotty and his group. They have studied long-term B cell memory after smallpox vaccination in a previously (3 months to 60 years) vaccinated group. Their results demonstrated initial exponential decay of memory B cells, with a half-life of <1 year, followed by a plateau ~10-fold lower than peak that is stably maintained for >50 years after vaccination [21]. Several studies also demonstrated that memory CD4+ and CD8+ T-cells to vaccinia antigen persist from months to decades after last smallpox revaccination [20–24]. Hsieh et al. showed that healthy subjects who were vaccinated within the last three decades and had a visible vaccination scar had remarkable T-cell reactivity compared to people who did not have a scar, or were vaccinated more than four decades ago [25].

Yet, the clinical significance of these studies in terms of protection against variola infection is not clear, and the exact level of immunity in the population today, 10–35 years after termination of continuous vaccination campaigns, is largely unknown.

Reference

1. Zilinskas RA, Hope B, North DW. A discussion of findings and their possible implications from a workshop on bioterrorism threat assessment and risk management. Risk Anal 2004; 24(4):901–908.
2. Haas CN. The role of risk analysis in understanding bioterrorism. Risk Anal 2002; 22(4):671–677.

3. Kwik G, Fitzgerald J, Inglesby TV, O'Toole T. Biosecurity: responsible stewardship of bioscience in an age of catastrophic terrorism. Biosecur Bioterror 2003; 1(1):27–35.
4. Atlas R, Campbell P, Cozzarelli NR, Curfman G, Enquist L, Fink G, et al. Statement on the consideration of biodefence and biosecurity. Nature 2003; 421(6925):771.
5. Sidel VW. Bioterrorism in the United States: a balanced assessment of risk and response. Med Confl Surviv 2003; 19(4):318–325.
6. Aragon TJ, Fernyak SE. The risks and benefits of pre-event smallpox vaccination: where you stand depends on where you sit. Ann Emerg Med 2003; 42(5):681–684.
7. Anand P. Public health. Decision-making when science is ambiguous. Science 2002; 295(5561):1839.
8. Karwa M, Currie B, Kvetan V. Bioterrorism: preparing for the impossible or the improbable. Crit Care Med 2005; 33(1 Suppl):S75–95.
9. Bozzette SA, Boer R, Bhatnagar V, Brower JL, Keeler EB, Morton SC, et al. A model for a smallpox-vaccination policy. N Engl J Med 2003; 348(5): 416–425.
10. Zubieta JC, Skinner R, Dean AG. Initiating informatics and GIS support for a field investigation of bioterrorism: the New Jersey anthrax experience. Int J Health Geogr 2003; 2(1):8.
11. Wagner MM, Dato V, Dowling JN, Allswede M. Representative threats for research in public health surveillance. J Biomed Inform 2003; 36(3):177–188.
12. Ferguson NM, Keeling MJ, Edmunds WJ, Gani R, Grenfell BT, Anderson RM, et al. Planning for smallpox outbreaks. Nature 2003; 425(6959):681–685.
13. Kaplan EH. Preventing second-generation infections in a smallpox bioterror attack. Epidemiology 2004; 15(3):264–270.
14. Schultz CH. Chinese curses, anthrax, and the risk of bioterrorism. Ann Emerg Med 2004; 43(3):329–332.
15. Fine AM, Wong JB, Fraser HS, Fleisher GR, Mandl KD. Is it influenza or anthrax? A decision analytic approach to the treatment of patients with influenza-like illnesses. Ann Emerg Med 2004; 43(3):318–328.
16. Alibek K. Smallpox: a disease and a weapon. Int J Infect Dis 2004; 8 (2 Suppl):S3–8.
17. Orr N, Forman M, Marcus H, Lustig S, Paran N, Grotto I, et al. Clinical and immune responses after revaccination of Israeli adults with the Lister strain of vaccinia virus. J Infect Dis 2004; 190(7):1295–1302.
18. Fenner F, World Health Organization. Smallpox and its eradication. Geneva: World Health Organization, 1988.
19. el-Ad B, Roth Y, Winder A, Tochner Z, Lublin-Tennenbaum T, Katz E, et al. The persistence of neutralizing antibodies after revaccination against smallpox. J Infect Dis 1990; 161(3):446–448.

20. Hammarlund E, Lewis MW, Hansen SG, Strelow LI, Nelson JA, Sexton GJ, et al. Duration of antiviral immunity after smallpox vaccination. Nat Med 2003; 9(9):1131–1137.
21. Crotty S, Felgner P, Davies H, Glidewell J, Villarreal L, Ahmed R. Cutting edge: long-term B cell memory in humans after smallpox vaccination. J Immunol 2003; 171(10):4969–4973.
22. Littaua RA, Takeda A, Cruz J, Ennis FA. Vaccinia virus-specific human CD4+ cytotoxic T-lymphocyte clones. J Virol 1992; 66(4):2274–2280.
23. Demkowicz WE, Jr., Littaua RA, Wang J, Ennis FA. Human cytotoxic T-cell memory: long-lived responses to vaccinia virus. J Virol 1996; 70(4):2627–2631.
24. Frelinger JA, Garba ML. Responses to smallpox vaccine. N Engl J Med 2002; 347(9):689–690.
25. Hsieh SM, Pan SC, Chen SY, Huang PF, Chang SC. Age distribution for T-cell reactivity to vaccinia virus in a healthy population. Clin Infect Dis 2004; 38(1):86–89.

SOME PUBLIC HEALTH PERSPECTIVES ON QUANTITATIVE RISK ASSESSMENTS FOR BIOTERRORISM

Steve Leach
Health Protection Agency, Centre for Emergency Preparedness and Response, Porton Down, Salisbury, Wilts, SP4 0JG, UK

1.   Background

In the context of bioterrorism and public health infrastructure public health professionals have a number of particular and crucial roles. These run in parallel with those in a wide range of other operational and strategic disciplines, such as those related to:

- More general national and international threat assessments
- The maintenance of local, national and international resilience
- The empowerment of emergency and essential services

Public health roles include assisting with the:

- Identification of potential threats (horizon scanning and surveillance)
- Formulation of policy
- Undertaking of planning
- Implementation of new, or the augmentation of existing, response capabilities

Under these headings potentially come:

- Improvements in diagnostics (detectors)
- The stockpiling of countermeasures, such as drugs and equipment
- The identification of existing and/or development of new systems for immediate response, and subsequent primary and secondary care (e.g., hospitals/treatment/decontamination centres),
- The clear delineation of lines of communication and data flows
- The training of responders

M.S. Green et al. (eds.), Risk Assessment and Risk Communication Strategies in Bioterrorism Preparedness, 19–29.
© 2007 *Springer.*

The public health process also involves assisting with:

- Raising and maintaining general awareness
- Testing and reviewing plans through desk-based and field exercises, and through these exercises
- Updating planning and policy

Many of these public health-related activities would also be common to preparedness for more natural emerging infectious disease threats, such as those posed by severe acute respiratory syndrome (SARS) and pandemic influenza.

2.   Different "Motivations" for Risk Assessment and Modeling

For the threats posed by both bioterrorism and "exotic" emerging infectious diseases the data and solid contemporary evidence-base on which to develop preparedness are usually limited or lacking. Further, and especially for communicable diseases, the emergent disease dynamics are also often likely to be nonlinear and frequently far from obvious because of the complexities and feedbacks in the disease and public health control mechanisms (Ferguson *et al.*, 2003). Models that accurately capture what evidence is available (often from historical data, laboratory experiments, etc.), therefore, often provide indispensable tools to investigate "what if" scenarios, examine alternatives control options, and develop policy and planning. A key benefit of using models to examine disease control options is their ability to explain and, with appropriate caveats and sensitivity analysis, predict trends at a population level from interactions and processes at the individual level. Models, however, have to be appropriately designed for the questions being addressed (Ferguson *et al.*, 2003).

Often, there are also useful distinctions that need to be made between the types of modeling that might be appropriate for more general threat-assessment exercises and those that might be required from a public health perspective. This can provide some interesting communication challenges. For example, the potential impacts of deliberate releases on public health and public health systems can be orders of magnitude greater than the impacts that might be identified by a more general threat assessment that is based on the more immediate or final effects, such as the likely numbers of directly attributable deaths. This is true of noncommunicable agents and even more so for communicable agents.

3.   Noncommunicable Agents – e.g., Anthrax

For example, for a simple estimation of the potential threat that might be posed by the deliberate release of a noncommunicable agent, such as anthrax, it might be sufficient to estimate the immediate number of casualties that might be caused by such a release, and compare these directly with the numbers of casualties that might be caused by other types of threat, such as an explosion or chemical incident. Typically for this, atmospheric dispersion and biological effects modeling would take into consideration such factors as the:

- Likely amount of material released
- Means of dispersal
- Particle size distribution
- Typical (or a range of) meteorological conditions for the area
- Underlying human population densities/distributions
- Typical breathing rate(s)
- Assumed dose/response relationship for the agent

There are considerable uncertainties in estimating much of the above, both from the perspective of the airborne dispersion modeling and, possibly more importantly, from the human effects modeling. In the case of the latter this arises because most of the information on which dose/response curves are based is derived from observations on animal species other than man and at high dosages. The latter are generally equal to or greater than the infectious dose 50% (ID_{50}) (or lethal dose 50% – LD_{50}), such that the effects of lower, but still pathogenically important, dosages have to be assumed from broad extrapolation.

On top of these uncertainties is compounded the issue that many more people would have been geographically situated so as to have been potentially exposed than would eventually be expected to succumb without treatment (Wein *et al.*, 2003). This has significant impacts from the point of view of estimating the public health difficulties that might arise from a deliberate release of a biological agent, and responding to it, compared to the basic estimation of the possible final casualties.

Depending on what is considered to be an acceptable risk in the underlying population, as against the uncertainties in determining that risk (e.g., as an illustration only, in Figure1, an $LD_{0.01}$ represents a 1 in a 10,000 risk of becoming infected and dying without treatment – and not assumed here to be an acceptable risk), then the numbers potentially exposed could be orders of magnitude higher than those that would be expected to succumb to that exposure. This point is elaborated upon later. Further, since it is unlikely to be possible to distinguish between those who have been potentially exposed and those who will then subsequently become ill, it will be necessary to find and treat as efficiently as possible all those who have been potentially exposed. In the case of anthrax this should ideally be done as rapidly as possible and before symptoms begin to show.

Figure 1 provides a very simple illustration of the above arguments (the values given on the axes are purely illustrative and based on a single hypothetical scenario – however, the approximate relationships shown are likely to hold over a considerable range of similar events). As the distance from the site of a release increases (x-axis) the probability of infection in those exposed decreases (related to the dosages of material to which they are exposed), but the numbers of individuals potentially exposed to the airborne dispersed pathogen are, to a first approximation, likely to increase roughly as the square of the distance (dashed line). This assumes a sufficiently even distribution of individuals on the ground over which the plume of material has passed (i.e., "the effective area of the plume at a given dosage contour"). Moreover, the numbers of individuals that are likely to become ill will increase much more slowly and approach a limiting value with distance.

The public health-related challenges are, therefore, to estimate how far from the release site the risk of becoming infected might be acceptable (and to whom amongst the various stakeholder groups such a risk is acceptable), and specifically identify the potentially large numbers of individuals that might have been exposed at this level of risk and deliver treatment to them quickly. Depending on the particular biological agent and the preferred treatment, this has also to be balanced against the possible risks (e.g., side effects) of giving the treatments themselves to an increasingly larger number of individuals, most of who would not have succumbed to the biological agent without treatment anyway. As is often the case with this type of activity, an overarching challenge is the clear communication of the potential implications of the uncertainty in such assessments and the factors that lead to those uncertainties.

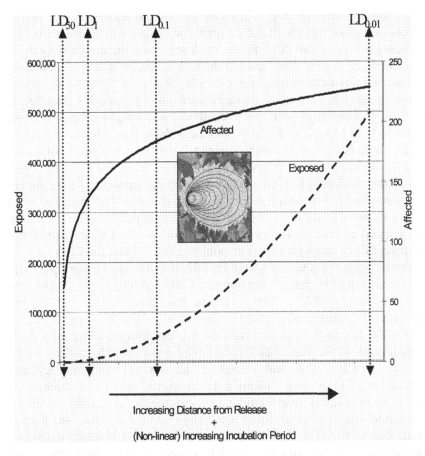

Figure 1. Showing, for a very hypothetical deliberate release, the relationships between distance from the point of the release and: the individual probability of infection and death without treatment for given dosages of pathogen potentially received (LD_n, vertical arrows, where n is the probability expressed as a percentage), the numbers of individuals exposed (dashed line) and the numbers affected (solid line). (Inset shows dosage contours LD_n over the ground for a hypothetical release over a population with varying density [thematically coloured]).

4.   Extending "Simple" Models for the Public Health Context

Public health contingency planning greatly benefits from combining the type of analysis described above for a whole range of deliberate release scenarios with other types of probabilistic individual-based risk assessment techniques. These need to take into account, for example, the time it takes to develop disease symptoms in those individuals exposed to different dosages of pathogen (which for anthrax can range from hours to weeks depending inversely, but not linearly, on dosage) and the time it is likely to take to find and deliver treatments to them. The results of such quantitative risk assessments demonstrate, for example, that even for anthrax, which at high dosages has a relatively short incubation period, it is feasible to find and successfully treat many of those who might otherwise have succumbed. In this case, for a hypothetical deliberate release over open terrain. There is, however, a very narrow window of opportunity following the deliberate release (or following the recognition of the first few cases after a covert release) in which it is necessary to mount a swift, efficient and appropriate public health response. This reinforces the perceived need to have in place good diagnostic and detection capabilities, as well as a well-planned emergency response infrastructure to rapidly deliver (ideally on a timescale of hours) appropriate public health countermeasures.

For "real-time" responses to covert releases, this type of pre-planning analysis also demonstrates that there are further public health challenges, since the first evidence that a release has taken place will be the appearance of individuals seeking medical help. On average, these are likely to be those that have received the highest dosages of the biological agent, nearest to the site of the release. The public health challenge here will be to rapidly link and recognize the unusual epidemiology and presentation of these cases, identify the biological agent and conduct in-depth epidemiological investigations to determine the geographic locations of affected individuals at times consistent with the likely incubation period distribution for the biological agent, which has been identified. Appropriate modeling strategies will then need to be rapidly applied to infer the likely location and extent of the prior initial release in order to find and administer treatment to those other individuals who have likely been exposed but have yet to develop symptoms. These will likely be those further from the site of the initial release, and who have received lower dosages than the initial cases. They are also likely to have the best prognosis following treatment if it can be delivered in time before symptoms develop. This again emphasizes the need to have in place good diagnostic and detection capabilities and well-planned and prepared emergency response infrastructures. These are required not only to deliver treatments, but also to develop and maintain enhanced public health awareness of the possible manifestation of "unusual" biological agents, as well as to promote the epidemiological and modeling techniques that will be required to identify those who need treatment.

5. Some Further Public Health Risk Assessment Issues for Communicable Agents

The public health impacts, and the response effort necessary to be put in place to mitigate or control them, can be even greater in both extent and duration for communicable agents. As sometimes done for more immediate, general, comparative threat assessments it might be (but is probably rarely) sufficient to simply compare the potential overall levels of initial mortality likely to be associated with a range of different initial release scenarios involving different types of agent. This, however, disregards the potential for onward transmission, the extent to which the initial threat might be amplified within the initially unexposed population, and the extent of the public health resources that would be required to bring a potential expanding epidemic under control. For public health contingency planning significantly more detailed modeling is required, to take into account levels of morbidity, as well as mortality, the dynamics of disease development in individuals and populations following exposure, as well as the numbers potentially exposed not only to the initial release but also as contacts of any ongoing infectious cases. Those initially exposed and requiring treatment will again number orders of magnitude higher than those who would be likely to eventually succumb. These numbers will also be considerably amplified as a consequence of the multiple contacts between infectious individuals and the rest of the previously unexposed population.

6. Pneumonic Plague

For example, this potential for amplification within the community has been examined using relatively simple individual-based stochastic models for the case of relatively small numbers of initially infected cases of pneumonic plague either accidentally introduced or deliberately caused within a population, without the knowledge or forewarning (i.e., covertly) of the affected community (Gani and Leach, 2004). Estimates of the extra burden that might occur due to the amplification of the initial release depend on the extent to which pneumonic plague is assumed to be transmissible from person to person. Analysis of historical data suggests that this (R_0) is low, with infected individuals on average infecting about one further person in the absence of public health interventions. The public health impacts also depend on the extent to which there is an alert, prompt and efficient public health response. If this response is efficient and effective, then for each initially infected person it is possible that there might only be on average between a further 1.5–3 cases caused by transmission within the community for each infection caused by the initial release itself. However, this could raise further to 4–10 more cases per initially infected case in more extreme examples. This situation could arise, either just by chance, and/or as a consequence of assuming values for R_0 (a measure of the transmission rate of pneumonic plague) at the higher end of the range that is supported by analysis of small historical data-sets.

Pneumonic plague has a rapid onset from infection and short time to death following symptoms. Symptomatic, infectious individuals are also typically extremely unwell and generally not ambulatory. Consequently, the prospects for infectious contacts are somewhat limited (hence the low estimates of R_0) and tended in the past to be in those family and health care workers who were looking after patients. In the case of health care workers, however, that was until such times as the disease was correctly diagnosed and nosocomial transmission eliminated. The prognosis for infected individuals given appropriate antibiotic treatment is also generally good, as are the prospects for the control of an outbreak. The latter is probably because the R_0 is low, cases only become infectious once they are symptomatic (and therefore more obvious), and thus the contacts of infectious cases are also likely to be easily identified. Nevertheless, the potential for ongoing person-to-person transmission for agents, such as plague within the community for some time following an initial release potentially adds to the other public health consequences and the burdens of a deliberate release that have already been discussed for anthrax. These will include an even closer epidemiological investigation of cases and the identification of their contacts, and the delivery of antibiotic treatments to an even larger number of individuals than those initially exposed to the deliberate release (i.e., to include all of the defined contacts of every case).

7.   Smallpox

Considerable risk assessment and modeling work has also been undertaken for deliberate releases of the communicable agent of smallpox. In this case, R_0 values, historically, were considerably higher than for pneumonic plague (Gani and Leach, 2001; Eichner and Dietz, 2003). This led some published assessments to conclude that mass vaccination was likely to be required to bring outbreaks under control most efficiently and reduce the extent to which the initial release was amplified in the community by person-to-person transmission (e.g., Kaplan et al., 2002). However, as stated earlier, it is necessary in these pre-planning risk assessments to take into account the extent to which there might be adverse events to vaccination and balance this against the extent to which possible epidemics would amplify in the community with more targeted vaccination and public health strategies (including, active case finding, contact tracing and isolation measures). More recent studies have suggested that more targeted approaches might be more appropriate (Eichner, 2003, Kretzschmar *et al.*, 2004, Eubank *et al.*, 2004). These depend to some extent on:

- The extent of the initial release (Kaplan, 2004)
- Whether the epidemiology of smallpox in a modern population can be reliably inferred from historical data (Ferguson *et al.*, 2003)
- Particularly with respect to, among a great number of other things, estimates of its transmissibility (R_0) and the associated contact patterns that would be relevant in contemporary communities
- The extent to which infected individuals might be infectious prior to symptoms becoming obvious (Fraser *et al.*, 2004)
- The extent to which public health measures, such as the isolation of cases and the monitoring of contacts, could be maintained (Kaplan *et al.*, 2003, Kaplan, 2004)

It will therefore be important in the early stages of an outbreak (and subsequently throughout it) to carefully monitor all aspects of its epidemiology and progress. This will require carefully planned systems of data collection, analysis and modeling, which raises further concerns that are particular to public health risk assessments and the estimation of the likely burdens that might be posed by deliberate releases of biological agents.

8.   Conclusions

In developing models for risk assessment, therefore, it is important to agree with those setting policy and drawing up plans the particular scope of the individual problem(s) that needs to be addressed and the applications that are anticipated for different models. It is also necessary to ensure that the public health and other responses that will be considered are feasible – an "ideal" public health solution that is not actually workable is rarely going to be helpful. It is also important to ensure that infectious disease and public health experts agree with the parameterizations and assumptions that are to go into modeling. It is also important that they are prepared to be flexible and responsive in the event of a real release to carefully reassess previous planning in the light of incoming epidemiological data and real-time data analysis and modeling. To achieve this it is important to engage as wide a range of stakeholders in the risk assessment process as possible and recognize that an iterative process is most likely to be necessary. An iterative process is also likely to be of greatest benefit and involve not only risk assessment, but also close linkages with risk management and communication. Indeed, to a considerable extent these activities should ideally be integrated at some level early on and maintained. This in itself can pose some interesting challenges because of the potential sensitivities associated with some of this work.

Acknowledgments

The author wishes to acknowledge the work and support of colleagues in the Health Protection Agency (HPA) (especially at Centre for Emergency Preparedness and Response – CEPR and Centre for Infections – CfI) and key UK academic collaborators (especially at Warwick University and Imperial College), and particularly the risk assessment team at CEPR (particularly Dr. Ray Gani). Aspects of this work have been supported by funding through the UK Department of Health, the UK Health Protection Agency and the EC Health and Consumer Protection DG (DG SANCO). The views expressed in the publication are those of the authors and not necessarily those of the Department of Health, the HPA or DG SANCO.

References

1. Eichner M, Dietz K. Transmission potential of smallpox: estimates based on detailed data from an outbreak. Am J Epidemiol 2003; 158: 110–117.
2. Eichner M. Case isolation and contact tracing can prevent the spread of smallpox. Am J Epidemiol 2003; 158: 118–128.
3. Eubank S, Guclu H, Kumar VS, Marathe MV, Srinivasan A, Toroczkai Z, Wang N. Modelling disease outbreaks in realistic urban social networks. Nature 2004; 429: 180–184.
4. Ferguson NM, Keeling MJ, Edmunds WJ, Gani R, Grenfell BT, Anderson RM, Leach S. Planning for smallpox outbreaks. Nature 2003; 425: 681–685.
5. Fraser C, Riley S, Anderson RM, Ferguson NM. Factors that make an infectious disease outbreak controllable. Proc Natl Acad Sci USA 2004; 101: 6146–6151.
6. Gani R, Leach S. Transmission potential of smallpox in contemporary populations. Nature 2001; 414: 748–751.
7. Gani R, Leach S. Epidemiologic determinants for modeling pneumonic plague outbreaks. Emerg Infect Dis 2004; 10: 608–614.

8. Kaplan EH, Craft DL, Wein LM. Emergency response to a smallpox attack: the case for mass vaccination. Proc Natl Acad Sci USA 2002; 99: 10935–10940.
9. Kaplan EH, Craft DL, Wein LM. Analyzing bioterror response logistics: the case of smallpox. Math Biosci 2003; 185: 33–72.
10. Kaplan EH. Preventing second-generation infections in a smallpox bioterror attack. Epidemiology 2004; 15: 264–270.
11. Kretzschmar M, van den Hof S, Wallinga J, van Wijngaarden J. Ring vaccination and smallpox control. Emerg Infect Dis 2004; 10: 832–841.
12. Wein LM, Craft DL, Kaplan EH. Emergency response to an anthrax attack. Proc Natl Acad Sci USA 2003; 100: 4346–4351.

SITUATIONAL AWARENESS IN A BIOTERROR ATTACK VIA PROBABILITY MODELING

Edward H. Kaplan
William N and Marie A Beach Professor of Management Sciences
Yale School of Management
Professor of Public Health
Yale School of Medicine
Professor of Engineering
Yale Faculty of Engineering

Johan Walden
Assistant Professor of Finance
Haas School of Business
University of California, Berkeley

1. Introduction

Following the events of September 11, 2001 and the subsequent anthrax mailings in the United States, the threat posed by bioterrorism has received renewed attention by governments across the globe. Though no large-scale attacks have occurred as of the date of this writing, several scenarios have been studied in detail, including deliberate releases of smallpox [1, 2], anthrax [3], plague [4], and botulinum [5], among others. While the specifics of these scenarios differ in terms of the dispersion mechanisms of the infectious agents and the resulting casualties that could result, all such analyses emphasize the importance of early detection and rapid response in mitigating the consequences of a bioterror attack.

There have been many different suggestions to detect a bioterror attack, ranging from the use of biosensors [6] to syndromic surveillance [7], to screening blood donors [8], to case identification. Once an attack has been detected and the agent has been identified, however, the key concerns become establishing the scale of the attack and forecasting how casualties will emerge over time. Such forecasts can guide the allocation of response resources; for example, is it necessary to add "surge capacity" to hospitals in the impacted area or are existing facilities adequate for expected caseloads. The real-time aspect of this approach enables rapid reassessment

31

M.S. Green et al. (eds.), Risk Assessment and Risk Communication Strategies in Bioterrorism Preparedness, 31–44.

of the situation as new caseload information arrives over time, and also provides useful guidance for deciding when the outbreak has ended (in the sense that few cases remain to be uncovered). We refer to such real-time monitoring, assessment, and forecasting activities as *situational awareness*.

This chapter illustrates the basic situational awareness problem with the aid of a recently developed model applied to a hypothetical anthrax bioterror attack [9]. The intent is to introduce the sorts of analyses that are possible using probability models that are simple enough to evaluate in an ordinary spreadsheet program such as Excel. Though some specific numerical assumptions will be made to provide a working example, the reader should focus on the nature of the information one could obtain from such methods rather than the specific numerical results that follow from the details of this example.

2.   The Situational Awareness Problem

Suppose that the first human case in a bioterror attack has just been observed, and that the agent involved has been determined. As more human cases are reported, it is critical to ascertain answers to two questions: how big was the attack (i.e., how many persons were infected); and when did it happen. The answers to these questions can then be used to create forecasts of future cases, which in turn can be used for emergency planning (e.g., is there sufficient hospital capacity to handle expected future cases, or is there a need for adding surge capacity). Estimates of the time and size of a bioterror attack also figure prominently in determining when the resulting outbreak has ended (i.e., when the expected number of future cases is very small compared to the estimated size of the outbreak). Additional situational awareness questions include establishing the location and spatial spread of an outbreak. Also, while this chapter will focus on techniques derived from observing human cases over time, one certainly could extend these ideas to attacks that are detected via biosensors, syndromic surveillance, or other means.

3.   An Anthrax Example and Attendant Assumptions

In the example to be developed, an anthrax attack infecting 100 persons has occurred. How will those infected in the attack reveal themselves over time? The key assumption employed is that the probability distribution of the *incubation time* from infection through the onset of symptoms is known.

Cases will thus appear in a manner consistent with this probability distribution. For anthrax, Brookmeyer et al. [10] studied the incubation time data associated with the Swerdlovsk accidental anthrax release and via maximum likelihood were able to fit a lognormal distribution with median 11 days and dispersion 2 days to the incubation time data associated with that outbreak. Figure 1 shows the lognormal probability density with the parameters stated above.

It is assumed that no interventions were launched prior to detecting the attack, which is reasonable: in the absence of any evidence of an attack, on what basis would one launch an intervention? However, while interventions might be launched once an attack has been detected (e.g., distribution of antibiotics to persons in the vicinity of the attack), it is further assumed that such interventions will not have any impact on the occurrence of cases during the first several days of the outbreak (as these cases would be among persons with sufficiently advanced infections to render intervention ineffective). Anthrax being a noncontagious agent, there will be no need to account for secondary transmission in our illustrative example. More complicated models allowing for secondary and continuing transmission (e.g., as would be the case with smallpox) can also be constructed, though such extensions will not be pursued in this chapter.

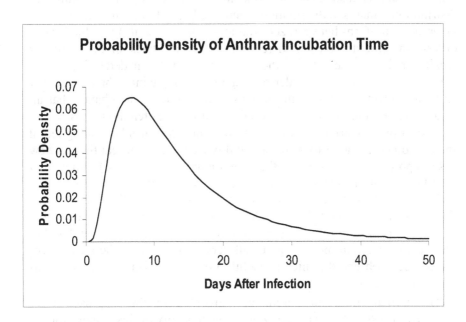

Figure 1. Probability density of anthrax incubation time.

4.   Basic Ideas

The key insight that enables one to estimate the time and size of a bio-terror attack from case reporting data is this: if n persons were infected in the attack, then the time from the attack until the 1st, 2nd, 3rd, ..., nth cases occur would be the *order statistics* from the incubation time distribution [11]. In particular, the time from the attack to the first observed case would correspond to the *minimum* of n independent incubation times (where the independence reasonably assumes that the progression of infection in any one individual has no influence on the progression of infection in any other individual). Thus, if one knew the size of the attack, one could estimate the time of the attack by working backwards from the time of the first observed case.

Of course, the size of the attack is not known, but it is possible to quantify prior beliefs regarding the likelihood that attacks infecting different numbers of individuals could occur. A Bayesian approach formally accomplishes this by postulating a prior probability distribution governing the size of the attack. Any such distribution should be diffuse to express our considerable ignorance over the likelihood that any one of a wide range of different attack sizes would occur. An attractive choice that satisfies this criterion and is also easy to work with is given by the log-uniform distribution – that is, a distribution where the logarithm of the attack size is taken to be uniform between zero (an attack size of unity) and the largest order-of-magnitude considered reasonable for an attack of this sort (for recall that it is assumed that the agent used has been determined; e.g., anthrax). This amounts to order-of-magnitude uncertainty: the chance that an attack infects a number in the tens is the same as the chance that an attack infects a number in the hundreds, thousands, or ten thousands.

Once a prior distribution for the initial attack size has been assigned, it then becomes a straightforward probability exercise to, in real time as new case reports arrive, estimate the conditional (or posterior) probability distributions of the attack size and time via Bayes' rule, given the number and timing of observed cases to date. Once armed with these conditional distributions, further probabilistic calculations enable a forecast of the number of cases expected in the future, as well as computation of the probability that at least a certain percentage of all persons infected in the attack have already been observed (which is useful in deciding when the outbreak has essentially ended).

The formal probability arguments involved in this approach were presented in [9] and are summarized in the appendix of this chapter for the technical reader. To show how such a model could be used in an actual bioterror attack, we return to our anthrax example and consider what might happen over the course of a single outbreak. Note that all of the calculations involved in this example were performed using an Excel spreadsheet, indicating the technical ease with which the models can be implemented [9].

5. A Simulated Example

Imagine that an anthrax attack occurs that infects 100 persons. The time from infection to symptoms follows the lognormal incubation time density of Figure 1. To obtain a specific example, 100 incubation times were randomly selected from this probability distribution and ordered to create the "actual" occurrence of cases over time (as reported on a daily basis) shown in Figure 2. Using the probability models proposed, it is possible to estimate the conditional probability distribution of the number infected in the attack given the cases observed to date since the detection of the attack. Figures 3–7 show this distribution having observed all cases through days 2, 5, 10, 20, and 50, respectively. From Figure 2, one can see that a total of 8, 25, 59, 80, and 100 cases were observed as of these dates. Note how the uncertainty in the attack size distribution disappears over time as more cases are reported, that is, how the probability densities increasingly place most of their weight on attack sizes in the vicinity of (the true value of) 100 as more information is collected. This illustrates how the model is able to "learn" from the data (and via the incubation time distribution) over time.

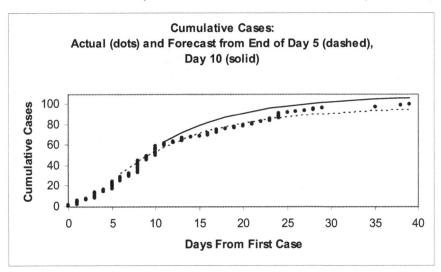

Figure 2. Cumulative actual and forecasted anthrax cases over time in the simulated outbreak.

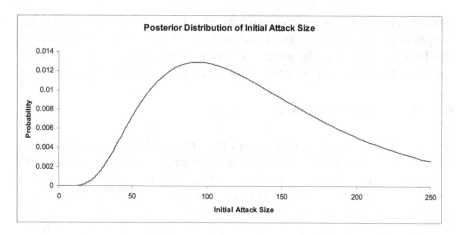

Figure 3. Attack size probability distribution 2 days after seeing the first case (Eight cases observed in total).

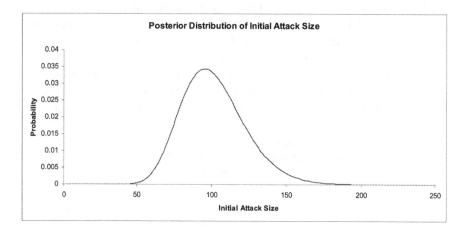

Figure 4. Attack size probability distribution 5 days after seeing the first case (25 cases observed in total).

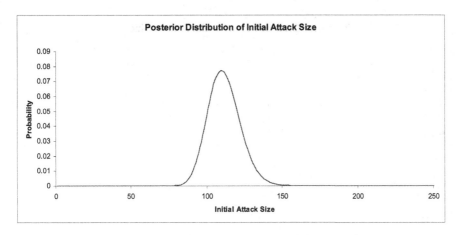

Figure 5. Attack size probability distribution 10 days after seeing the first case (59 cases observed in total).

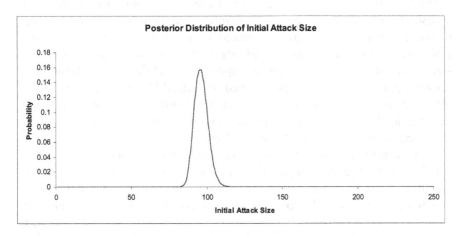

Figure 6. Attack size probability distribution 20 days after seeing the first case (80 cases observed in total).

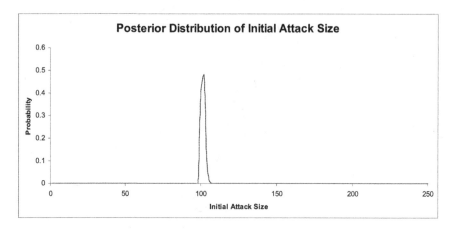

Figure 7. Attack size probability distribution 50 days after seeing the first case (100 cases observed in total).

While Figures 3–7 reveal that considerable "learning" occurs over the course of this simulated outbreak, it is interesting that the mean attack size (a point estimate as it were) computed from these distributions as new information arrives over time is quite stable. Figure 8 plots the mean attack size as estimated over time from the updated probability distributions, and shows that the point estimates obtained do indeed hover closely about the true value of 100. One would expect accurate estimates once most of those infected in the attack have progressed to symptoms, but Figure 8 shows that good results are obtained much earlier.

Considerably less information is gained regarding the timing of the attack. Figures 9 and 10 report the probability distribution of the time of the attack as measured in days prior to observing the first case after days 2 and 50 of the outbreak. In both cases the bulk of the probability locates the attack to have occurred between 1 and 3 days before the first case was observed. The information gained from day 2 to day 50 essentially rules out the possibility that the attack occurred more than 3 days prior to the date of the first case.

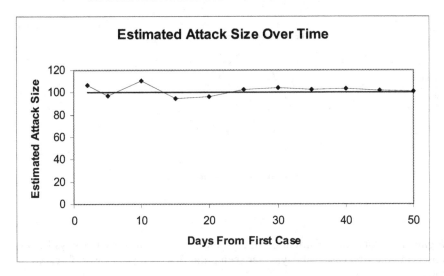

Figure 8. Expected (mean) attack size as estimated over time from detection of the outbreak from the first observed case.

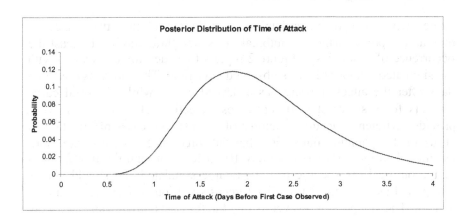

Figure 9. Probability distribution of the time of attack (measured as days before observing the first case) 2 days after seeing the first case (Eight cases observed in total).

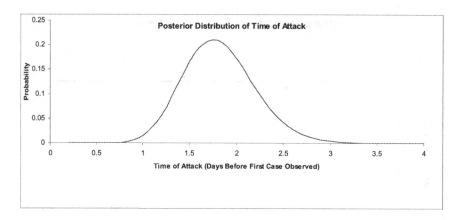

Figure 10. Probability distribution of the time of attack (measured as days before observing the first case) 50 days after seeing the first case (100 cases observed in total).

6.   Forecasting Future Cases

Armed with the updated probability distributions of the attack size and time at any point during the outbreak, it is straightforward to forecast the occurrence of future cases. Figure 2 reports two such forecasts along with the simulated number of cases observed over time. The forecasts created 5 days after the attack appeared as a dashed curve, while the solid curve presents forecasts created 10 days post-detection. Both these forecasts provide sufficiently accurate pictures of downstream cases of infection to be useful for planning purposes. That the forecasts from day 5 are more accurate than the forecasts from day 10 (at least through the first 24 days of the outbreak) is specific to the example simulated and should not be interpreted as meaning that earlier forecasts will outperform later ones in general. The key point, however, is that the forecasts provide an early view of how those infected in the attack will reveal themselves over time, enabling appropriate planning for care and treatment to ensue early in the outbreak.

7.   Is the Outbreak Over?

Thus far the focus has been on estimating the time and size of a bioterror attack in order to predict future caseloads. However, whether or not to declare that an outbreak has ended is also a crucial decision. Brookmeyer and You [12] proposed a statistical hypothesis test based on the spacing between observed cases for deciding whether an outbreak has ended. An alternative approach follows directly from the Bayesian principles employed in the present chapter. Specifically, one can calculate the probability that at least $100\alpha\%$ of *all* cases have been observed at any point during the outbreak (and for any value of α). For example, one can compute the probability that at least half of all cases have already occurred as of the date of computation, or if at least 80%, 95%, or even 100% of all cases have occurred. The probability that at least $100\alpha\%$ of all cases have been observed is referred to as the α-level outbreak completion probability.

Figure 11 plots α-level outbreak completion probabilities for $\alpha = 0.5$, 0.75, 0.95, and 1 for the data in our simulated anthrax attack. Note that one is about 80% certain that at least half of all cases have occurred after day 10 of the outbreak (and indeed, 59 cases already occurred by day 10, which is more than 50% of 100, the true number infected in the outbreak). It of course takes longer for the outbreak completion probabilities to approach unity as α increases; it requires 80 days and 100 observed cases (which in the example constitute *all* of the cases that could occur) to be 95% certain that the outbreak is over (i.e., the α-level outbreak completion probability equals 95% for $\alpha = 1$ only after 80 days). The method is thus appropriately conservative when asked if the outbreak is truly over.

Outbreak Completion Probability

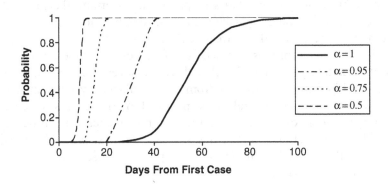

Figure 11. α-level outbreak completion probabilities over time.

8. Summary

This chapter has provided a simple example showing how one can use the probability distribution governing the incubation time from infection through symptoms for a bioterror agent with observed cases in real time to estimate the time and size of a bioterror attack, forecast the number of downstream cases for planning purposes, and assess over time the extent to which the outbreak is totally or partially complete. The computations required can be carried out in an Excel spreadsheet [9], as was all of the computing for the example presented.

While it is hoped that that this chapter serves to convince the reader of the value of probability modeling in bioterror preparedness and response, the methods and example presented are not the final word on this subject. This chapter has only concerned itself with a noncontagious bioterror agent such as anthrax. Attack with a contagious agent such as smallpox, plague, or tularemia would require additional modeling to account for continuing transmission from those initially infected; deconvolution methods similar to the back calculation of human immunodeficiency virus (HIV) incidence from acquired immunodeficiency syndrome (AIDS) reporting data would be required [13]. The approach has also assumed that the incubation time probability distribution is known, but while information is available for many feared bioterror agents [14], it might be that for either new or modified viral or bacterial infections, the data observed in the outbreak itself becomes the best information describing incubation times (as was the case with the accidental release of anthrax in Swerdlovsk [10]). In this instance, it would be possible to augment the modeling approach suggested to account for uncertainty in the incubation time distribution, and to statistically update this distribution and hence learn in real time as those infected present themselves as cases. However, although it is not difficult in principle, loss of precision governing the incubation time distribution would translate to considerable loss in precision regarding the forecasts of downstream cases.

Finally, the model proposed based all inferences over time on observed cases of infection, yet as noted earlier there are several proposals, such as the use of biosensors and/or syndromic surveillance systems meant to speed the detection and general assessment of bioterror events. It remains to integrate models of the form reported in this chapter with those other more elaborate detection and reporting systems; doing so would be a major advance in the provision of decision support to those concerned with managing the consequences of a bioterror attack.

References

1. Kaplan EH, Craft DL, Wein LM. Emergency response to a smallpox attack: the case for mass vaccination. Proc Natl Acad Sci USA 2002; 99:10935–10940.
2. Halloran ME, Longini IM, Nizam A, Yang Y. Containing bioterrorist smallpox. Science 2003; 298:1428–1432.
3. Wein LM, Craft DL, Kaplan EH. Emergency response to an anthrax attack. Proc Natl Acad Sci USA 2003; 100:4346–4351.

4. Gani R, Leach S. Epidemiologic determinants for modeling pneumonic plague outbreaks. Emerg Infect Dis 2004; 10:608–614.
5. Wein LM, Liu Y. Analyzing a bioterror attack on the food supply: the case of botulinum toxin in milk. Proc Natl Acad Sci USA 2005; 102:9984–9989.
6. Estacio, PL. Bio-Watch Overview. Washington, DC: Department of Homeland Security, 2004. Available at: https://www.nlectc.org/training/nij2004/estacio.pdf
7. Das D, Metzger K, Heffernan R, Balter S, Weiss D, Mostashari F. New York City Department of Health and Mental Hygiene. Monitoring over-the-counter medication sales for early detection of disease outbreaks – New York City. MMWR Morb Mortal Wkly Rep 2005; 54(Suppl):41–46.
8. Kaplan EH, Patton CA, FitzGerald WP, Wein LM. Detecting bioterror attacks by screening blood donors: a best-case analysis. Emerg Infect Dis 2003; 9:909–914.
9. Walden J, Kaplan EH. Estimating time and size of bioterror attack. Emerg Infect Dis 2004; 10:1202–1205.
10. Brookmeyer R, Blades N, Hugh-Jones M, Henderson DA. The statistical analysis of truncated data: application to the Swerdlovsk anthrax outbreak. Biostatistics 2001; 2:233–247.
11. David HA. Order statistics. New York: Wiley, 1970.
12. Brookmeyer R, You X. A hypothesis test for the end of a common source outbreak. Biometrics 2005 (online early, doi:10.1111/j.1541-0420.2005.00421.x).
13. Brookmeyer R, Gail MH. AIDS Epidemiology: A Quantitative Approach. New York: Oxford University Press, 1994.
14. Centers for Disease Control and Prevention. Biological agents/diseases: category A. Atlanta (GA): The Centers, 2003. Available at: http://www.bt.cdc.gov/agent/agentlist-category.asp#a

Appendix

This appendix summarizes the formulas used in the models of this chapter. For greater detail please consult [9]. The analysis centers on two random variables, the number infected in the attack N, and the time of the attack (measured as time before the first observed case) A. The probability distribution of the incubation time from infection through symptoms is assumed known, and in particular the probability that an incubation time exceeds x is denoted by the survivor distribution $S(x)$.

Suppose that the attack size $N = n$. Since the attack is detected by the first observed case, the probability density of the time of attack given $N = n$ is given by

$$f(a \mid n) = nS(a)^{n-1} f(a) \quad \text{for} \quad a > 0, n = 1,2,3,\dots \tag{1}$$

If the prior probability distribution for the attack size is given by $p(n) = \Pr\{N = n\}$, then the joint probability distribution of the attack time and size is given by

$$f(a,n) = p(n) \times nS(a)^{n-1} f(a) \quad \text{for } a > 0, n = 1,2,3,... \tag{2}$$

Now, suppose that by time τ, an additional $k-1$ cases have been observed beyond the initial case observed at time 0 that signaled the outbreak. Conditional on the attack size $N = n$ and the attack time $A =$ (days before observing the first case), the probability of observing these additional cases at times $t_2, t_3 \ldots t_k \leq \tau$ (where $t_1 = 0$ denotes the time at which the first case is observed) is given by

$$\mathsf{L}(\mathbf{t}\,|\,a,n,\tau) = \frac{(n-1)!}{(n-k)!} \left\{ \frac{S(a+\tau)}{S(a)} \right\}^{n-k} \prod_{j=2}^{k} \left\{ \frac{f(a+t_j)}{S(a)} \right\} \tag{3}$$

The joint probability of observing $N = n$, $A = a$, and the data actually seen then equals

$$J(a,n,\mathbf{t}\,|\,\tau) = p(n)\frac{n!}{(n-k)!} S(a+\tau)^{n-k} \prod_{j=1}^{k} f(a+t_j) \quad \text{for } a > 0, n = k, k+1, k+2... \tag{4}$$

Bayes' rule then implies that the conditional probability distribution of the attack time and size given the data observed up to time τ after the attack was detected is given by

$$f(a,n\,|\,\mathbf{t},\tau) = \frac{p(n)\dfrac{n!}{(n-k)!} S(a+\tau)^{n-k} \displaystyle\prod_{j=1}^{k} f(a+t_j)}{\displaystyle\sum_{i=k}^{\infty} \int_{u=0}^{\infty} p(i)\dfrac{i!}{(i-k)!} S(u+\tau)^{i-k} \prod_{j=1}^{k} f(u+t_j)\, du} \quad \text{for } a > 0, n = k, k+1,... \tag{5}$$

All of the quantities of interest can be computed from Equation (5). For example the α-outbreak completion probabilities can be computed as

$$\Pr\{\frac{k}{N} \geq \alpha \,|\, \mathbf{t},\tau\} = \sum_{n=k}^{\lfloor k/\alpha \rfloor} \int_{a=0}^{\infty} f(a,n\,|\,\mathbf{t},\tau)da \quad \text{for } 0 < \alpha < 1 \tag{6}$$

Details for computing forecasts of future cases and other quantities can be found in [9].

THE BIOTERRORISM THREAT

Yair Sharan
The Interdisciplinary Center for Technological Analysis and Forecasting at Tel-Aviv University, Israel

Non-state actors have caused significant economic and psychological damage using chemical and biological agents. Fortunately, such events have been rare; none very successful, and all have resulted in few casualties. Nonconventional weapons in the hand of terrorists are more properly termed "weapons of mass impact" rather than weapons of "mass casualties."

Most analysts perceive bioterrorism as highly probable, easy to achieve, and likely to cause a huge number of casualties. The Biothreat picture has been fueled by "hysterical" predictions of natural outbreaks of very deadly diseases such as smallpox, Ebola, and Marburg, and threat assessments that tend to the extreme. The reality is that terrorism has achieved more with conventional means; terrorists apparently question the value of bioterrorism. The seemingly incongruous terrorist behavior has a strong rationale. A rigorous technical evaluation (Sharan et al., 2000) uncovers the difficulties terrorists have trying to achieve a biological weapon (BW) capability.

The present paper gives a balanced picture of the bioterror threat and discusses the impediments to non-state actors attempting to achieve this capability.

1. Threat Assessment

Inclusion of BWs in a terrorist arsenal reduces to two questions: (1) can the weapons be acquired from a nation state – legally or otherwise or (2) can the terrorist group itself develop the weapons. The issue has been discussed extensively. The first is a political issue; development is a technical matter.

Most analysts seek analogies to determine feasibility for such weapon acquisition and reach conclusions based on appreciation of the technical capabilities of industrialized countries. Such analyses commonly foresee

M.S. Green et al. (eds.), Risk Assessment and Risk Communication Strategies in Bioterrorism Preparedness, 45–54.
© 2007 *Springer.*

nonconventional weapons as attainable by terrorist groups and their use likely in the future. Those assessments also forecast mass casualties.

This chapter develops a new perspective for assessing future terrorist capabilities. Our analysis is consistent with past Network Centric Warfare (NCW) experiences – particularly the terror events in Japan in the early 1990s and the US September 11 events. It presents a more realistic appreciation of future capabilities and effects.

2.   General Analysis

Our objective is to determine whether a terrorist group can develop a capability through its own efforts. Our approach identifies and analyzes the technical requirements needed to develop BW and establishes whether the technology is within the grasp of a terrorist organization. We find some elements in the BW development process currently doable, some only possible after a huge investment, and others not likely to be mastered in the foreseeable future.

An advantage of our approach is that the focus on separate technical steps allows identification of critical thresholds, telltales, and formulation of proactive and reactive defense measures.

Figure 1 illustrates a BW development program. It breaks the development process into seven steps beginning with acquisition of the basic knowledge to the actual weapon use. Specific steps include operation choice, acquisition of critical equipment and weapon components, manufacture, weaponization of the agent, storage and transport of agents and the weapon during manufacture, and finally weapon use in the field. The process is highly visible in less-developed countries and more easily hidden in a highly industrialized country.

We have applied parallel versions of Figure 1 to the development of chemical, nuclear, and radiological weapons. To test the methodology, we recruited a highly trained technical chemist with an MSc degree (Sharan et al., 2000) and tasked him to design a chemical weapon, identify in detail the equipment needed and production protocols, and describe all telltales that would expose such a clandestine program. The exercise underscored the difficulties in translating theory to weapons. Moreover, it highlighted the dangers involved in producing and handling lethal materials. Manufacturing techniques and dangers are never fully discussed in the open literature. Mistakes are generally catastrophic. This kind of *Gedanken* experiment resulted in weapons of low quality and pointed out critical steps

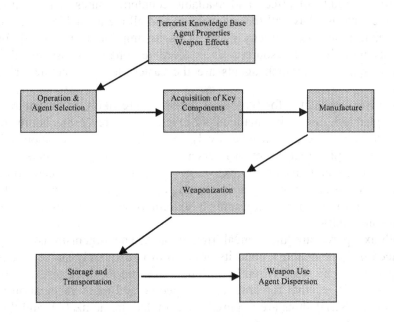

Figure 1. Technical steps for terrorist development of nonconventional weapons.

and thus guidelines for detection and defense. The same principles apply to nuclear and BWs.

3.   Knowledge Gathering

The first step is for terrorists to develop a knowledge base about different agents, their properties and potential danger to people. It is widely held that a simple literature and Internet search are sufficient and a capability could be easily achieved. This is an exaggeration. The distance from theory to application in this case is enormous even if the literature is complete in all details which it is not (Meselson, 1999).

4.   Agent Selection

Biological agents can be selected according to several considerations such as toxicity, resistance, disease contagiousness, their lethal versus incapacitating properties, rapidity of effect, and available countermeasures. This is true when the terrorists have all the information and all the available means to produce, test, and deliver any agent. This assumption is not valid for terrorists with limited resources. It is more reasonable to assume that selection reduces to which agents are the easiest to manufacture or to obtain.

The main candidates for biological terrorism are likely to be anthrax, plague, glanders, tularemia, smallpox, T2 mycotoxin, Q fever, and botulism. All those agents have been extensively researched, several weaponized, and some (despite treaty) remain in arsenals. Some biological agents may be aerosolized and dispersed over large area; some agents and some diseases such as smallpox or plague spread person to person. The ability to infect beyond the primary exposures is extremely worrisome in a mobile global community.

Anthrax spores are the logical first choice. The organism is easily produced in large quantities and its dried form is extremely stable. It has been produced and weaponized by different labs and its characteristics are well-known. It is lethal for unvaccinated people and mass vaccination is problematic. Serial shots are required for complete immunization and this requires complicated logistical preparations.

Smallpox is highly contagious and infectious among unvaccinated people and no specific treatment exists. Because routine vaccination stopped 20 years ago, only a small fraction of the population has immunity. Smallpox could be introduced by terrorists that illegally obtain agents from repositories in the United States, Russia, or other unregistered sources. *Plague* is attractive to terrorists, because it may continue to spread in the population after the initial aerosol dissemination. Plague is also easily spread by infected vectors. Plague is however unstable at high temperature and in sunlight. In climates similar to Israel or California the spread effectiveness is low.

Tularemia is another disease that could be chosen by terrorists to be disseminated during an attack, especially because it is a lethal agent and is infectious at lower dosage than anthrax. It is a persistent lethal contaminant and viable for weeks in water.

Two toxins that could be selected by terrorists are those that cause botulism and mycotoxins. Botulinum toxin is the most toxic compound known to man and readily extracted from *Bacillus* and *Clostridium botulinum* cultures. There is evidence that T2 mycotoxin was used in the past.

5.   Acquisition

There are several modes of acquisition of biological agents that could be used by terrorists:

- The primitive way – using a natural contagious source (e.g., ill people, corpses, and endemic sites)
- Self-production after mastering the needed technologies
- Theft of agents from research labs
- Theft of biological munitions held by military forces
- Receipt of ready-made BWs from a sponsor state

We concentrate on self-production or collection from natural sources.

Biological agents are very much correlated to modern microbiology. The development of biological agents as weapons has paralleled advances in basic and applied microbiology. This includes the basic knowledge that can enable identification of virulent pathogens suitable for aerosol delivery, and industrial-scale fermentation processes that produce large quantities of pathogens and toxins.

Any modestly sophisticated pharmaceutical or fermentation industry with mass production capability for growing cultures used in commercial production of yeast, yogurt, beer, antibiotics, and vaccines may be a candidate – If accessed by terrorists – for producing pathogenic microorganisms. Almost all the equipment needed for the production of pathogens and toxins is dual-use and available on the international market. The potential for hiding illegal activities under the cover of legitimate production is real and worrisome. Small quantities of botulinum toxin, for example, is used as a drug for treatment of disabling diseases and for cosmetic applications.

In a short time, a lab could be cleared of all suspicious material and look like any medical or pharmaceutical research lab. (Contamination however is likely to remain and be detectable.) Sterile work and even mass production of organisms can be done on a relatively small scale. A seed culture of anthrax bacteria could be grown to mass quantities in weeks. Most of the required production techniques are described in textbooks and journals. Production though is extremely hazardous, and cleanup – while straightforward – is strenuous and requires rigorous safety protocols.

Advanced biological technologies have spread all over the world. There is a large pool of highly trained "bio" personal, and methods for culturing large quantities of bacteria are well known. "It is impossible to tell whether biological research is intended for purposes of warfare until an actual agent is used. Some agents that can be used for biological warfare are also used

for peaceful purposes. There is nothing that is so deeply dual-use"
(Lederberg, 1997).

While national and international conventions restrict availability of
agents, the system is not foolproof. For example, in March 1995, Larry
Harris, a microbiologist and a member of the Aryan Nations used a forged
letterhead to order samples of *Yersinia pestis*, the organism that causes
plague, from the American type culture collection (ATCC) in Rockville,
Maryland. He was caught only when it was found that he did not have the
special equipment needed to handle the organisms. The anthrax used in the
envelope events in the United States after 9/11 apparently involved weapon
grade agent.

Sites in Africa, for example, where frequent outbreaks of contagious
disease have occurred could be of high interest to terrorist groups seeking
starter cultures. Some events are shown in Table 1.

TABLE 1. The African supermarket – recent outbreaks in Africa (From Dr. Julius
Julian Lutwama, *Viruses in Uganda*)

Year	Disease	Country
1992–1993	Yellow fever	Kenya
1995	Ebola	Congo
1998	Rift Valley fever	Kenya, Uganda
1999–2000	Marbury	Congo
2000–2001	Ebola	Uganda
2003	Yellow fever	Sudan
2004	Ebola	Sudan

Undergraduate microbiology skills can be used to isolate *B. anthracis*
from cattle, where the disease is endemic. Using this as the starter culture,
in a few days a terrorist could brew several kilograms of crude slurry
containing billions of spores in a 100-L vessel. Drying the slurry for dry
agent production is tricky, though not impossible. Freeze drying, in which
material is frozen and put under vacuum to remove water, is one option.
Grinding the (slurry) powder into micron-size particles is a key challenge,
mainly because of the risk of contamination and infection. A much easier
approach could be to use a wet slurry agent, which when applied, will
result in smaller numbers of casualties.

The Aum Shinrikyo cult that released the chemical agent Sarin in the
Tokyo subway had a surprisingly well-developed technical infrastructure
for chemical and of BWs (Kaplan, 1997). This included front companies
for purchasing materials and equipment, well-equipped laboratories and

extensive chemical and biological manufacturing facilities. They had more than 40,000 members and one billion dollars in assets. The cult had a large BWs program. As early as 1990, they were trying to aerosolize botulinum toxin. They attended unsuccessfully to harvest bacteria in Africa and in an expedition to Zaire they tried to obtain samples of the Ebola virus. So far, the substantial Aum program has not resulted in a BW arsenal. Cases in which anthrax was released in Tokyo caused no casualties as the agent was far below weapon standard (despite a reasonably effective dispersion). The difficulty to realize a BW capability is further shown in the case of Iraq.

Evidence from the Iraq BW program shows the complexity of producing and weaponizing BW agents. Contrary to their successful chemical weapon program, the Iraqis failed to produce effective BWs. In the light of the relatively non-impressive results, it is probable that for non-state groups it will be even harder to succeed.

In conclusion, several routes of acquisition are open for terrorists to try and produce bio-agents by themselves. Some routes can be blocked by an effective international system, which denies access to available sources by unauthorized people. Better inspection of relevant labs and industries will also help. We expect that availability of agents in the future to terrorists will be more difficult and self-development and production will remain very problematic.

6. Storage and Transportation

Special training and equipment is needed to store and transport biological agents safely. This is a severe impediment to most terrorist groups. Freeze-dried storage is one preferred way to store biological agents for a long time. However freeze-drying an agent is not trivial, and more resources and skills, than those generally available to terrorists are needed.

7. Weapons Use and Methods of Delivery

There are several means by which terrorists could try to deliver BW agents:

- Dispersal via air within enclosed or open areas
- Transmission through infected vectors such as fleas, ticks, flies, or rats
- Contamination of foodstuffs or liquids at their source or during production or distribution

BW agents are nonvolatile particulates disseminated either as liquid slurry, or a dry powder of freeze-dried organisms or toxins in aerosols. Possible delivery systems range in complexity and effectiveness from simple agricultural sprayers, up to specialized cluster warheads, carried by ballistic missiles.

A key factor in producing large-scale respiratory infections is the ability to generate a stable aerosol cloud of suspended microscopic droplets, containing from one to thousands of bacterial or viral particles. Effective respiratory infection of man requires dispersal of particles smaller than 10 μm. Small particles settle in the lower respiratory tract while larger particles are filtered or expelled by the body, although they still contaminate the environment creating a secondary health threat.

Dissemination of biological agents using conventional munitions seems a simply dispersion technique, but it has certain technological difficulties and limitations because most biological agents are sensitive to explosive environments and further more are destroyed by environmental stresses such as ultraviolet (UV) radiation, humidity, and oxidation.

Weather is another important consideration. High wind speeds tend to break up aerosol clouds. Rain or snow scavenges most aerosols from the atmosphere. Inversion conditions and low wind speeds (5–20 km/h) which occur more often during nighttime and in early morning hours are ideal conditions for biological agent dispersal.

Aerosols also may be produced by industrial sprayers with nozzles modified to generate smaller drop sizes. The aerosol could be dispersed along a line using an airplane or boat traveling upwind of the intended target, or from point sources using stationary sprayers. More sophisticated delivery systems could use missiles, dispensing agent-containing bomblets in areas upwind of a target, or spraying the agent from flying platforms (aircraft or unmanned aerial vehicles [UAVs]).

A commercial aerosol disperser mounted on a truck or a car, could be used by terrorists to attack a city with biological agents. A quick Internet search reveals a wide range of agricultural sprayers and foggers. The quality of the equipment is surprisingly high and relatively cheap. A typical sprayer weighs 6 kg, costs about $350, and disperses particles in the range of 7–30 μ. Such equipment could achieve efficiencies of 10% and more (some claim even 50%) based on inhalation of droplets or particles of diameter less than 10 μm.

Although manufacture of a BW capable of causing mass casualties is not trivial; the effective delivery of a BW agent by terrorists is most likely even more problematic.

Many analysts point out that biological agents could be used to poison reservoirs supplying drinking water. Many of the highly lethal biological agents are not effectively transmitted by water and are neutralized by chlorination and water purification processes. Contamination of a municipal water supply requires compensation for a significant dilution and hence very large quantities of biological agent are needed. So much so that terrorists would find acquisition, transport, and dumping of such mass quantifies far too difficult. Israel's water network is well protected by systems which would "detect" such hazardous events.

Food is vulnerable to contamination by terrorists. Biological agents could be inserted into production lines turning out packaged prepared food or in bulk foodstuff or beverages. However, past events like the poisoning of Israeli oranges or the dioxin food contamination in Belgium show that casualties are limited and that the health system is quick to respond to such events. The main effect is extreme public anxiety.

8. Casualty Assessment

Because biological agents are lethal in very small quantities, many sources in the literature estimate millions of casualties as a result of a BW attack on an unprotected population. However, such estimates are often based simply on the minimum lethal dose under optimal dispersion conditions. Lethality figures drop sharply, when factors such as agent concentration, population density, and practical dispersion characteristics under realistic conditions are taken into account.

Analyses (Purver, 1995) show that 50 kg of anthrax spores introduced into the air-conditioning system of a domed stadium could infect 70,000–80,000 spectators within 1 h.

OTA (1992) estimated the casualties from delivery of anthrax spores by a Scud-type missile and dispersal by a single aircraft. In the first case, 30 kg of the agent caused 30,000–100,000 casualties, and 50 kg in the second mode caused 420,000–1,400,000 casualties. Those calculations use simple dispersion models and assume a "medium" case of overcast weather and moderate winds. On clear windy days the estimated number of casualties would be lower; on clear calm nights, the estimated number of casualties would be higher. Based on such estimates, OTA concluded that pound for pound, BWs such as anthrax, plague, tularemia, and botulism could exceed the killing power of nuclear weapons. We note though that ideal dispersion conditions rarely persist long enough to achieve the situations required to support those casualty estimates and that (despite the low weights) extremely large amounts of agent are being deployed. Moreover, the calculation assumes an agent quality and amount that is most unlikely that a terrorist group to immobilize and deploy.

We developed four basic scenarios (Sharan et al., 2000) for realistic estimates of casualties and size of the area affected by a terrorist biological attack. The agent – consistent with a clandestine ad hoc effort – is a crude solution of cultivated anthrax, with a concentration of 10^{11} spores/L. This concentration represents that achievable by terrorists with little experience and low-tech lab or production equipment. For all risk estimates, we assume that the effective dose is 10^4 spores (inhaled). The breathing rate is fixed at 15 L/min corresponding to people occupied in mild office activities.

An attack on a closed theater seating 300 people results in exposure of most is virtually people in high dosages ranging from a few to tens of ED_{50} depending on the effectiveness of the disseminator. An attack in an open area in which anthrax is dispersed using point source explosion results in far fewer casualties.

A detailed simulation (Sharan et al., 2000) of a container of 10–24 kg of liquid anthrax exploding in the center of Tel-Aviv with 1% dispersion efficiency would cause between 10 and 90 casualties comparable to attack with conventional explosives. More casualties are expected if that amount of anthrax would be continuously dispersed from a fixed sprayer in a congested area. The number of casualties can reach several thousands depending on the weather conditions and time of attack.

9.   Conclusions

In our work, we have directed the nonconventional weapon production process to realistically assess the threat of bioterrorism. In contrast to "conventional wisdom", we found that development and use of BWs is far from trivial and in most cases presents almost insurmountable obstacles to terrorist groups. Redirect estimates of casualties resulting from an attack by bioterrorists show in several scenarios effect of the order of a conventional event questioning the wisdom of use of such weapons. This does not reduce the need for vigilance and precaution, but does offer a more realistic assessment of risk.

References

1. Kaplan DE. The cult at the end of the world. New York: Crown Publishers, 1997.
2. Lederberg J. Infectious disease and biological weapons: prophylaxis and mitigation. JAMA 1997; 278:435.
3. Meselson M. The problem of biological weapons. Private communication, April 1999.
4. Sharan Y, Small R, et al. Non-conventional terrorism. June 2000, 191 p. E/107.
5. OTA. Technology against terrorism: structuring security. United States Congress, Office of Technology Assessment, Washington, DC, 1992.
6. Purver R. Chemical and biological terrorism – the threat according to the open literature. Canadian Security Intelligence Service, 1995. http://www.csis-scrs.gc.ca/eng/miscdocs/purve.html

CHANGE OF MIND-SET FOLLOWING 9/11: THE FEW THAT ARE ALREADY WILLING TO RESORT TO WEAPONS OF MASS DESTRUCTION

Yoram Schweitzer
*Associate Researcher for INSS (Institute for National
Security Studies).*
www.LABAT.co.il

The 9/11 attack in the United States was unequivocally a formative event in the history of modern international terrorism, with a major effect on the characteristics of terrorist activity in the international arena.[1] The anthrax attacks in the United States following the 9/11 attack, albeit not considered part of the Global Jihad terror campaign, aggravated the fear that we were at the beginning of a new era and in the midst of an all out war by all means available. Indeed what we have heard after the 9/11 and even more so following the counterattack by the US coalition in Afghanistan and later in Iraq is willingness to breach all the taboos, by at least **some** elements within the Global Jihad camp. Given the chance and means they will use every weapon, including weapon of mass destruction, they can lay their hands on, in order to badly hurt their declared enemies headed by the United States.

---

[1] Yoram Schweitzer, Shaul Shay. An expected surprise: the September 11th attack and its ramifications. Herzliya: Mifalot Publishing. The Interdisciplinary Center, 2002, p. 15 (Hebrew); English version forthcoming in June 2003: The globalization of terror: the challenge of al-Qaeda and the response of the international community. New Jersey: Transaction Publishers, Rutgers University Press, pp. 49–52.

*M.S. Green et al. (eds.), Risk Assessment and Risk Communication Strategies in Bioterrorism
Preparedness, 55–66.*

1.   Terrorism – Essentially a Psychological Weapon

Terrorism of any kind involves hurting people in order to frighten a much larger audience than the specific attacked target, and thereby influence through tactics of societal fear the political process. In considering the use by terrorists of weapons of mass destruction (WMD) we must keep in mind and not further exacerbate the existing societal fears that terrorists are already using to manipulate the public. Therefore, it is essential to define our terms carefully. Conventionally, WMD denote ominous weapons that up to very recently were only in the domain of states and had the potential to kill thousands and many more. We should not lump together under this category smaller-scale potential attacks with radiological, chemical, or BWs and more lethal types of BWs and nuclear arms since their potential to harm is not the same.

In the analysis of a nonconventional terrorists threat one has to bear in mind that we need to make a clear distinction between the various types of nonconventional weapons available to terrorists: chemical, radiological, biological, and nuclear (CBRN). Nuclear terrorism bears the most lethal threat which can be evaluated in terms of thousands of fatalities to hundreds of thousands and even more with additional catastrophic maladies like cancer and other kinds of injury as well as long-lasting environmental damage. Terrorism involving biological materials as well can cause high numbers of fatalities, epidemics, and contamination of areas and wide collateral damage. Chemical terrorism (and some biological attacks as well, e.g., ricin) are highly dependent on the quantity, quality, weather conditions, and the way it is dispersed and brought to its target. Radiological terrorism, as opposed to the use of nuclear weapons can cause fatalities and contamination of a very limited area, but its main effect will be psychological. This is true of chemical and some biological terrorism as well. Thus, we see devastating results if nuclear and some biological terrorism is engaged and much more limited lethality, but profound psychological impact and media attraction in the case of chemical, radiological, and some biological types of attacks.

2.   Organizational Concerns in the use of Weapons of Mass Destruction

We must also distinguish between the groups and networks that may resort to these weapons from the majority who will probably be reluctant to use them. Most of the terror groups which are operative today will likely refrain from resorting to such weapons as their ideology is to play within the system and not against its existence. They have a desire to not only survive but also obtain achievable political goals from the system and to get their share of power and ultimately become political actors within the system.[2] On the fringe of these groups there are a few groups and networks belonging to the Global Jihad led by al-Qaeda or closely associated with its ideas that have other ideological considerations and especially after 9/11 who perceive the conflict in terms of a zero-sum game. They are willing to go to any lengths to achieve their objective of total societal and political change. Yet, even in the circles of Global Jihad there are still groups that albeit their Islamic perceptions have a lot to loose and will probably not resort to WMD. Thus, there is a need to distinguish the specific ideological extremist groups like al-Qaeda and Zarqawi and his associates from the rest.

While trying to evaluate the potential risk of the various terror groups that may resort to the use of nonconventional materials and even more of WMD we should present some of the restraining factors that terror organizations take into consideration in the process of their decision making before choosing their targets and weaponry. Most terror organizations are inclined to refrain from steps that will alienate their constituency as they are looking for their support and usually also aspire to have international support for their group and actions in order to capitalize on it to exert pressure on the adversary government. In many cases terror organizations have a sponsoring state, whose broader and strategic considerations must be included in their decisions to act or to refrain from action or at least in the type of attacks they can carry out. These kinds of considerations have been playing a major role in the reluctance of terror organizations to engage in using nonconventional materials and surely WMD.

Most of the terror groups in the world today have clear political agendas and specific demands and considerations that are influenced by their goals, but at the same time they want to preserve their survivability.[3] However, there are several organizations with ideological extremist perceptions that are ready to be destroyed in the process of destroying others as they believe that God will provide for them in the afterlife.

---

[2] Anat Kurz. Non-conventional terrorism: availability and motivation. TAU Strategic Assessment, 7(4), March 2005.

[3] Ibid.

3.   Groups Considerations and their Probable use of Weapons of Mass Destruction

Groups considerations	Organization with high probability for using NCW	Organization with low probability for using NCW
Need for acknowledgment	Jihad Ideology/international/ nihilistic	The organization is seeking acknowledgment for its existence as well as for its demands
Organizational survivability	Organizational survivability is not crucial. The organizational structure is diffused and therefore flexible	Organizational survivability is an upper value
State dependency	The organization is not dependent on the support of the state	The organization is very dependent on the support of the state
Organization's need for international/local support	Nor local or international support is of importance to the organization	The organization gives high importance to both international and local support
Direct confrontations	Direct confrontations is a strategy for recruiting new members to the organization	The organization is refraining from direct confrontation

4.   Who are the Groups that may Resort to using Weapons of Mass Destruction?

Al-Qaeda and some close affiliates like Zarqawi and his associates are definitely looking for a full confrontation with all the means that they possess. This has become clearer after 9/11 and more so after the counterattack by the international coalition in Afghanistan and in the battle in Iraq as of mid-2003, as will be discussed more fully below.

Networks that operate under al-Qaeda's inspiration and in some cases with its assistance (direct and indirect) are difficult to deter as they tend to operate and then disintegrate and re-form in the future so their survivability as an existing organ has less importance for them and they do not exist as tangible targets to be attacked or have vested interests to be compromised. Indeed, it appears that the leaders of such networks often operate in an ad hoc manner forming groups that consume their members (as "martyrs") while their leaders disappear and reemerge in future to direct new operations on behalf of their ultimate mission of bringing about a new world order. This form of an "organization" does not have any tangible assets that can be attacked or a conspicuous Achilles' heel to step on in order to deter it so the only option is to find and destroy. That is exactly what makes this kind of networks so problematic to deal with in the "conventional" means used vis-à-vis the "normative" terror organizations.

5.   Lessons from Recent Chemical and Biological Attacks

To date the world has witnessed at least one notorious case where Aum Shinrikio (Supreme Truth), a nihilistic sect used both chemical and biological material in terror attacks in Japan in 1994 and 1995. Of these, the deadliest one was perpetrated in Tokyo in 1995 and involved releasing Sarin nerve gas, which killed a dozen of Japanese and injured hundreds going to hospital with minor symptoms. These attacks resulted in relatively low number of casualties and were not emulated by other organizations. The reasons may lie in the fact that they did not succeed in killing a stunning unusual number of casualties that is necessary to give a nonconventional material the appeal of a mega-terror instrument and hence failed any gains both from public support and building up the power image of the group. The lack of the global dimension as for example al-Qaeda and its associates have seems to be the crucial factor in its limited effect. The Aum Shinrikio had no connections with like minded groups in the world and lack the transnational mechanism to spread the psychological warfare that would give it the extra effect which usually utilized by the perpetrators to install fear in the targeted population. This may also have had something to do with that the group lacks a coherent political agenda and is much more cultish and Armageddon aimed than wanting political concessions from government. The fact that they failed to have a profound impact has likely made these types of attacks less attractive to those who might chose to emulate them. Thus, although the attack in Japan was the focus of considerable media coverage, as well as many academic studies and articles, because of its pioneering stature, it remained an exceptional, marginal phenomenon that was not imitated by other terrorist organizations.

Following 9/11 attack a small quantity of anthrax was disseminated in the United States by an unidentified sender who likewise failed to cause a high number of casualties but succeeded in inflicting a lot of panic in the American public and confusion in the administration that was enough to set up a national alarm towards the need to stand up to confront the challenge of biological warfare.

6.   9/11 – A Change in Consciousness within the Global Terror Organizations

Since the end of the 1960s, when modern international terrorism began playing an increasingly influential role in international relations, a large number of terrorist attacks have been carried out around the world. Only a small number yielded highly lethal results, killing dozens and in rare cases hundreds of people. Exceptionally, severe attacks were carried out infrequently, typically by different organizations and at significant intervals. Airplanes provided a ready venue for such attacks: 329 people were killed by the explosion of an Air India plane by Sikh terrorists in June 1985, and 270 people were killed in December 1988 when a Pan Am plane exploded over Lockerbie, Scotland, the work of Libyan agents. In some instances, car bombs loaded with thousands of kilograms of explosives and driven by suicide bombers were used to carry out attacks with mass casualties. The two terrorist attacks against United States Marines and a multinational French force in Beirut carried out by the Hizbollah in October 1983, which killed a total of almost 300 people, serve as primary examples of such attacks.

However, mass-casualty attacks killing thousands of people have only been planned and attempted by terrorist groups that are Afghan alumni, led by Bin Laden and functioning under the auspices of al-Qaeda. According to the Afghan alumni's increasingly extremist religious messianic world-view, the indiscriminate killing of large numbers of people is permitted, and even desirable, when it is done "in the path of god" (*"fi sabil Allah"*).[4] They interpret such acts as consistent with the commandments of the Koran and Islamic law. In this context, the transition to carrying out mega-terror attacks can be seen as a "natural" outcome of the cultural–religious confrontation between them and those whom they perceive as infidels, chiefly, in their terms, the "Judeo–Crusader alliance." Still, they do not refrain from the indiscriminate killing of others, such as Hindus in Kashmir and even "infidel" Muslims in Arab countries.

---

[4] Reuven Paz. YES to WMD: The first Islamist *Fatwah* on the use of weapons of mass destruction. PRISM Series of Special Dispatches on Global Jihad, 1, May 2003.

September 11, with its score of more than 3,000 deaths, heavy economic damage, and dramatization of American vulnerability, was an important morale-boosting victory for the Afghan alumni. It also represented a new, higher minimum standard in escalating terror attacks, as their architects work towards actualizing their vision of liberating Islamic holy lands and establishing an Islamic caliphate throughout the world.

Today, 5 years after September 11, one can discern an increase in intensity and frequency in the planning and execution of mass-casualty terror attacks, which reflects the profound change of consciousness that has taken place at the level of violence sanctioned, if not encouraged, in the struggle against infidels. *Accordingly, we have already reached the initial and in this case accelerated phase of the age of nonconventional terrorism.*[5] The Afghan alumni regard mega-terror attacks, whether using materials of conventional or nonconventional warfare, as legitimate. The execution of such attacks is primarily a function of the terrorists' performance capabilities, and timing is usually determined by their degree of operational preparedness and their overall operational strategy of maximizing the economic and psychological damage to their adversaries.

7.   Preparations for Using Nonconventional Weapons

Armed with extremist ideology and an agenda of indiscriminately killing their enemies in masses, the Afghan alumni's escalation within the international terrorism arena during the 1990s led them almost naturally to invest efforts in acquiring nonconventional weapons. Bin Laden's unequivocal 1999 statement that he regards the acquisition of such weapons as mandatory and as a religious commandment only increased fears that the day would soon come that this threat would be transformed from the potential to the actual. The US attack on the Shifa pharmaceutical factory in Sudan, which was suspected of producing chemical substances for al-Qaeda, lent credibility to the threat. Another expression of senior al-Qaeda leaders regarding nonconventional terrorism was the September 2002 television interview granted by Khaled Sheikh Mohammad to the television program *Sirri l'il-Ghaya* ("top secret"),[6] broadcast on

---

[5] Schweitzer Yoram. The age of non-conventional terrorism. TAU Strategic Assessment, 6(1), May 2003.

[6] Fouda, Yosri, and Nick Fielding. Masterminds of Terror: The Truth Behind the Most Devastating Terrorist Attack the World Has Ever Seen. New York: Arcade Publishing, 2003.

Al Jazeera. Khaled Sheikh, who supervised the 9/11 attack and was later arrested in early March 2003 in Pakistan, acknowledged that one of the directions considered by al-Qaeda on the eve of the 9/11 was an attack on a nuclear reactor in the United States. At the time the idea was rejected out of apparent concern that a successful attack of this nature would unleash uncontainable consequences and events would rapidly spiral out of control. Since then, hesitations of this sort appear to have abated.

The attack in Afghanistan uncovered numerous documents and extensive photographic documentation of training camps and hideouts of al-Qaeda members in Afghanistan. This documentation indicated the readiness of al-Qaeda and its affiliates to use nonconventional materials in terrorist attacks aimed at killing thousands of people. The most chilling documentation was broadcast on CNN in August 2002, showing the experimental use of poisonous substances on dogs in training camps in Afghanistan. This documentation can be added to the testimony of arrested al-Qaeda members such as Ahmed Rassem (arrested while attempting to smuggle weapons from Canada to the northwestern United States, as part of his plan to blow up the Los Angeles airport on the eve of the new millennium), who at his trial acknowledged that he and his colleagues underwent training with poisonous substances.

In addition, a number of events took place since September 11 that are likely to help and accelerate the formation of a "consciousness environment" supportive of the Afghan alumni's desire to use nonconventional warfare substances in their terrorist attacks.

- The explosion at the chemical factory in Toulouse, France, in September 2001 appears to have been caused by an act of sabotage carried out by a French Islamist of North African descent hired by the factory just a few days before the explosion. The incident caused the death of 29 people, as well as serious environmental damage. The French authorities went to great lengths to keep the incident quiet, among other reasons in order to prevent it from becoming a model for imitation.

- While the anthrax attack carried out in the United States shortly after the 9/11 attack appears to have been an act of protest most likely by an American scientist with no al-Qaeda involvement, it played a significant role in raising the standard of nonconventional operations, from chemical terrorism to biological terrorism. Despite the relatively small number of casualties caused by only a miniscule quantity of anthrax, the attack functioned primarily to highlight the potential of environmental damage and the blow to morale that a terrorist weapon of this sort can wield.

- The May 2002 arrest of Jose Padillia, an American citizen who converted to Islam, was trained in Afghanistan by al-Qaeda, and was sent by the organization to assess the possibilities of purchasing radiological material to detonate a "dirty bomb" in the United States, is also evidence of the operational directions of al-Qaeda in this realm.

- The assassination of Hatab, a prominent leader of Chechneyan terrorist organizations, with a poisonous substance concealed inside an envelope resulted in Chechneyan threats of taking revenge against the Russians in the same manner. Moreover, the Russian security forces' use of fentanyl gas while storming the Moscow theater caused the immediate paralysis and eventual death of many of the captors and the hostages. This was perceived by the Chechneyans as an act of escalation, accelerating the nonconventional phase in their own struggle against the Russians. Indeed, a terrorist cell arrested in France at the end of 2002 had planned a revenge attack against Russian targets in Europe using nonconventional materials.

- The arrest of al-Qaeda and its affiliated cells in various countries throughout Europe in early 2003[7] involved the January discovery in England of ricin (apparently only a small portion of a much larger quantity that had disappeared). A similar find occurred in March in France. These events reinforce the suspicion that al-Qaeda and the organizations it supports are preparing to wage nonconventional terror campaigns.

- The death of many al-Qaeda members, including some senior leaders and members of their families (e.g., the wife and daughters of Dr. Aymen al-Zawahir, Bin Laden's deputy), enhances the Afghan alumni's already radical worldview with the dimension of personal revenge. This is likely to dispel any moral inhibitions that still remained regarding the use of all warfare materials at their disposal and motivate them to execute terrorist attacks that are much deadlier than the one the world witnessed on September 11, 2001.

- The war in Iraq which added thousands of casualties to the accumulated count of Bin Laden while articulation of the justifications for future vengeance against the Americans and their allies by nonconventional means.

---

[7] Amit Cohen, Daphna Vardi. Europe under threat. Maariv supplement, 7 February 2003, 22–23 (Hebrew).

8.   The Race to the End

There are clear indications of al-Qaeda's efforts to obtain and produce components of NCW and Bin Laden public declaration that obtaining NCW capabilities is a religious duty gave it official posture. Indeed it seems that previously Bin Laden decided to refrain from attacking a nuclear plant in the United States: as he was reluctant, at that stage, to suffer the probable consequences. Following 9/11 the mind-set of Bin Laden and al-Qaeda changed regarding the use of nonconventional means including nuclear, given the chance they can obtain one.

The main reasons for this change in ideology and practice include [5]

- Al-Qaeda and its disciples worldwide were intoxicated by the success of the 9/11 attack.
- They were likewise enraged by the American aggressive response in Afghanistan and now Iraq.
- In consequence they turned to a "zero-sum game" mood.
- They elevated the level of violence in their planned attacks.
- A religious edict (fatwa) was issued to support the use of WMD which made it religiously sanctified. [8]
- This was followed by criticism by leading ideological figures regarding the previous practice of refraining from using WMD against the enemies. This criticism was mainly by Abu Musaab Al-Suri. In December 2004, Abu Musaab Al-Suri, a veteran and a prominent figure in the grand al-Qaeda ranks who published a 1,600 page book advocating a new organization of Global Jihad called "The Islamists Global Resistance." In this book that was issued on the Islamic circulated websites he outlined his strategy of Global Jihad. In this document he called for the use of WMD as an effective and necessary weapon against the enemies of Islam. He criticized Osama Bin Laden for not having previously used nonconventional weapon referring to Bin Laden reluctance to attack an atomic site as part of the 9/11 campaign. [9]

---

[8] Paz R. YES to WMD: the first Islamist *Fatwah* on the use of weapons of mass destruction. PRISM Series of Special Dispatches on Global Jihad, 1, May 2003.

[9] Paz R. Global Jihad and WMD: between martyrdom and mass destruction. Current Trends in Islamist Ideology 2005; 2, 74–86.

Due to the change in the character of the battle in the eyes of al-Qaeda and its closest allies and especially the ongoing bloody conflict in Iraq, the pretext for killing thousands and hundreds of thousands of Kafirs (apostates) among the "enemies of Islam" is permissible and even desirable.

Therefore, one can assume that

- Al-Qaeda and some of its affiliated networks are the primary candidates for resorting to the use of nonconventional materials in terror attacks; if they acquire them, they will be used under the right circumstances.
- Since religious approval has already been issued, the "justification" will be forthcoming.
- A breach of the "alleged taboo" and the copycat nature of terrorism may signal a start of a new era in global terrorism and it may either grow gradually to the level of small samples of nonconventional "soft" materials that will be used in sporadic attacks or that a major leap will be made by one group or network that will resort to more lethal materials and by that open a Pandora box which will cause an irretrievable tragedy.

The first step towards such developments must be to realize that the state of mind of such attack has already been around so it is more a matter of when, by whom, and at what level it may occur rather than if. The big race now is to prevent the Jihadists or any like-minded from putting their hands on a BW or more alarmingly a nuclear device.

9.   Summary

One of the most significant impacts of the 9/11 attack on global terror organizations has been the creation of a fundamental change in the consciousness of the mainly Afghan alumni-led al-Qaeda and some of its closest affiliated networks. The unprecedented success of the 9/11 attack created a sense of omnipotence among al-Qaeda and its supporters and encouragement to continue in this path. On the other hand, the US massive reaction in Afghanistan and Iraq backed by the international coalition enraged them and gave an impetus to their desire to take revenge against their declared enemies. This change has been reflected not only by the deeds, but also by the rhetoric of terrorist organizations' spokespersons, which may also signal a further escalation in the activity and readiness of some terrorist organizations to move forward into the "nonconventional terrorism era." Nonconventional terrorism that we can expect to see in the future may be characterized on two levels of activity. The first is small-scale use of chemical, and radiological and even biological weapons whose impact is primarily psychological in nature. The second level involves executing a monumental attack(s) "mega-terrorism" using nonconventional warfare materials in order to harm large numbers of people, cause long-term environmental damage, and deliver a public psychological and morale-crushing blow of a scope hitherto unknown. Thus, we find that in the period that has followed the 9/11 attack, that the standard of violence in terrorism has been increased significantly. The number and frequency of "high casualties" attacks planned or executed has been raised and the "taboo" surrounding terror "tolerated" lethality has likewise been removed. In contrast, and perhaps ironically, the public and the decision makers of the Western world have not experienced a change in consciousness regarding the nature of the threat and its degree of acuteness. Such a change, however, is essential to achieving the public support for an antiterrorism strategy that can adequately and effectively address the current terrorist threat. The race is on and we wait to see who will win.

ANTIMICROBIAL PROPHYLAXIS AND PROVIDING SUBACUTE CARE IN THE CONTEXT OF A BIOTERRORISM EVENT: LESSONS LEARNED FROM 2001

Jonathan Zenilman
Professor of Medicine
Division of Infection Diseases
John Hopkin University School of Medicine

1. Introduction

Since 2001, development of bioterror response capacity has largely focused on emergency management, development of diagnostic tools and algorithms, and ensuring capacity for acute care of casualties [1, 2]. This has included assuring supply of antimicrobials, vaccines, critical equipment, and hospital preparedness planning. The 2001 anthrax attacks demonstrated that *subacute response*, the ability of public health to mobilize screening, treatment, and dispensing capacity to large numbers of potentially exposed persons, was the major need. Despite this experience, there has been little planning for subacute response capacity.

In the context of a bioterrorism event, subacute response is providing assessment services, counseling, preventive treatment, and follow up to persons with potential exposure, and who are not clinically ill. Preparing the subacute response poses enormous logistical challenges. In most cities, providers of preventive health services, for example, municipal health departments currently provide only minimal clinical services, and have little surge capacity. Therefore, careful planning is critical.

This is a national problem. McGugh reviewed preparedness in 12 US metropolitan areas in 2002–2003 [3]. The vast majority of activity was in emergency preparedness/response activities and hospital preparedness. Major activities included increased disease surveillance, laboratory capacity, information and system technology, education, and workforce training (mostly for immediate disaster response). Challenges identified in this review were funding shortfalls, local budget deficits (independent of preparedness), which limited surge capacity, communications, and infor-

M.S. Green et al. (eds.), Risk Assessment and Risk Communication Strategies in Bioterrorism Preparedness, 67–76.

mation technology infrastructure, and public health staffing. "Respondents in some communities reported difficulties in hiring qualified public health workers, particularly nurses and epidemiologists, because of short supply and inability to offer salaries competitive with the private sector."

During the 2001 anthrax attacks, the health departments in the New York and Washington areas were presented with an enormous challenge; providing therapeutic treatment, preventive treatment, and counseling to thousands of individuals who were potentially exposed. This presented enormous stresses to the local health departments, but also presented opportunities for planning these types of events in the future. Their experiences have been extensively reviewed [4–8]. In reviewing the experience, it appears that the bulk of *all* clinical activities responding to the attacks were provided by direct health-care providers providing subacute care. Acute care hospitals, first responders, and emergency departments played only a minor role. This review will synthesize the reported literature reports, and the Baltimore Health Department experience of the 2001 outbreak, which addressed the subacute outpatient response.

In the United States, the structure of the public health system is highly decentralized – providing both major advantages and disadvantages for disaster planning. Public health in the United States is a local and state function specifically delegated as such in the US Constitution. Each of the 50 states has a health department, and within those states, there are a total of 3,100 local health departments, mostly at the county or municipal level. Over two-thirds of these departments serve small populations (less than 50,000 individuals) and have less than seven direct employees. Because of changes in the US public health system over the past decades, the clinical capacitiy of the public health system has actually decreased. Rarely do public health departments provide direct clinical services in primary care, and typically they are limited to areas which have public health impact, specifically those mentioned above. For example, health departments used to provide large amounts of primary pediatric and prenatal care. However, with expansion of managed care organizations, and provision of insurance to children and pregnant women, the need for public health provision of those clinical services has declined.

The published literature identifies five major problem areas in the 2001 anthrax attack response, and has been most comprehensively reviewed by Gursky [2], and critiques published by the US Government General Accounting Office [1]. These include:

1. *Communication* to public and private health providers. Health providers were presented with different exposure/treatment algorithms and advice from different sources. For example, in Maryland, Virginia, and the District of Columbia, each of the three state jurisdictions and the CDC all provided different levels, amounts, and quality of information. Groups such as Johns Hopkins University, in turn developed protocols and algorithms, specifically to address the absence of information; however, these bodies were not subject to any specific authority or regulation.

2. *Environmental testing.* Each of the different geographical areas had different protocols for environmental testing and development of treatment protocols for environmental exposure. These variations led to discontent, an even charges of racial discrimination. For example, different exposure treatment protocols were applied in the exposures at the US Senate and at the Washington post office, due to different jurisdictional authority, and differences in the type of exposure initially suspected. Because of the different socioeconomic classes and even racial/ethnic groups of the employees, the post office employees and their union later criticized the differential response.

3. *Ambiguous public health authority.* During the attacks, the public health authority to investigate, treat, and manage the outbreaks was somewhat ambiguous. There are multiple levels of governmental authorities, which were involved, multiple jurisdictions ranging from the county, city, and federal agencies, also involved were federal emergency management agencies, and the criminal investigative authorities at the state and local level.

4. *Coexistent criminal investigation.* Early on, it became very clear that the anthrax attacks were criminally motivated; therefore, the Federal Bureau of Investigation (FBI) and local police agencies became involved. Since the attack sites were defined as crime scenes, law enforcement authorities had primary responsibility. In some cases, there were delays in the sharing of information. Furthermore, the cultures between public health and criminal investigation authorities are substantially different with regard to information provision. This experience has resulted in development of cooperative joint public health–law enforcement task forces for bioterrorism attack response and investigation.

5. *Procurement.* Demand for antimicrobials, e.g., ciprofloxacin, far outstripped the supplies available in the public health departments, hospitals, and pharmacies. Despite that availability of the national emergency stockpiles, there is need for planning for the interim period before the stockpile supplies become available (typically 24 hours).

Despite these issues, the anthrax response did require substantial rapid mobilization of clinical and public health resources on a level not seen in the United States for decades. This involved rapid assessment teams, environmental assessment teams, as well as mobilization of staff and supplies required to provide clinical care and treatment to tens of thousands of exposed individuals. In contrast to outbreaks, which require vaccination or short-term prophylaxis, the anthrax treatment response required a long-term course of (60 days) of antibiotics [9, 10]. There were little data on the use of long-term antibiotics in such a large number of individuals, as well as the associated problems and questions regarding compliance, behavioral aspects related to compliance, and potential side effects. There were a large number of exposed and treated individuals. This pool continually expanded, as a result of decisions, which were made (which may or may not be a problem in and of itself) that basically provided treatment to any individuals who were potentially exposed. Because so little was known about the infectivity and spread of the anthrax in the letters mailed to the post office and to the individual offices, as the infectivity became more widely known, more individuals became eligible for treatment.

In essence all individuals who requested treatment were essentially treated. For example, in New York City alone 7,076 postal workers, and an additional 3,600 media and hospital workers were screened and offered treatment [5, 8]. In Washington, DC an estimated 3,400 persons were screened and treated [4]. These are probably underestimates, because there may have been individuals who were treated and not appropriately documented.

2. The Baltimore Experience

Our experience in Baltimore was illustrative. Baltimore is located 40 miles (67 km) north of Washington DC, and is considered as part of the Washington metropolitan planning area. On October 24, 2001, the Baltimore City Health Department (BCHD) was notified that 4,000 individuals would require treatment for being exposed potentially to anthrax. These were predominantly employees of local mail processing facilities and credit card payment processors, all of whom received mail from the impacted main post office ("Brentwood") facility in Washington. The initial request from the CDC came on a Wednesday afternoon, and it was anticipated that clinical facilities would be in place within 24 hours to initiate treatment, counseling, and public health prophylaxis.

The BCHD response utilized existing clinical personnel and facilities at the two health centers, which house the sexually transmitted diseases

(STD) and tuberculosis (TB) clinics, and field health services staff. Besides the clinic facilities themselves, three field clinics were also established within 24 hours at three public schools. Five days later one employer-based clinic was also established. This employer was a large credit-card payment processor with 400 employees.

The STD/TB clinic staff was utilized because they are employees with experience providing outpatient counseling, assessment, and clinical services under a variety of nontraditional conditions. Public health clinicians in Baltimore are nurse-practitioners and certified physician assistants working under the supervision of a physician. Their clinical expertise includes acute disease diagnosis and management, and providing treatment to exposure contacts.

Public health registrars are experienced at rapid intake procedures, including enquiring about relevant contact information. Public health disease intervention specialists are well acquainted with counseling functions, and also are able to provide field information and operate independently in field settings. Counselors and social workers, who are part of the human immunodeficiency virus (HIV) management team, were mobilized to assist in counseling individuals who may be under stress because of the events that were taking place.

Clinical protocols were rapidly developed with a partnership between health departments' senior leadership staff, infectious disease personnel from the Johns Hopkins University School of Medicine, the medical directors of the STD, TB, and HIV control programs, as well as nursing and emergency management staff. All protocols were developed in close consultation with existing clinical protocols available from the CDC, the Maryland State Department of Health and Mental Hygiene, and the Johns Hopkins University Infectious Disease Division.

The field clinics were set up with multiple stations. An intake registration station was staffed by disease intervention specialists and registrars. Patients were then directed to the assessment station, where they were examined by clinicians and provided with drugs. There was no dispensing pharmacist on-site; health department personnel were authorized to dispense the antibiotics under the emergency provisions. Physician supervision was provided onsite, and also by radio/mobile phone contact by infectious disease physicians and health department senior staff. Mental health counseling resources were available at all operating clinical sites and were provided by social workers. During this period of time standard STD, TB, and family planning activities were suspended for 4 days because of the intense resources allocated to these tasks.

One of the initial concerns at the beginning was drug procurement. Although ciprofloxacin was on formulary at the STD clinics, this is typically used as a single dose regimen. Therefore, initially, it would have been difficult to provide all patients requiring this medication with enough medication to last a 60-day course. Provisions were made for emergency procurement from the city health departments' supplier, and additional resources were identified in other communities, approximately 1 hour away. Arrangements were made for the Baltimore Police Department to provide emergency escort in case that was needed (in order to provide rapid supply). However, because of the rapid availability of the national stockpile supplies, drug supplies were adequate after the first day of operation. In Baltimore, over 2,500 individuals received preventive treatment in the 4 days of operation (Baltimore City Health Department, unpublished data).

3.   Resources that can be Mobilized

Public health clinicians and disease outreach staff are typically assigned to traditional clinical activities, which are almost exclusively performed by public health departments. These are STDs, TB management, family planning, and immunization and refugee health activities. These are the only direct clinical care employees employed by health departments. Because of their experience with field outreach, these classes of employees (public health nurses, physicians, interviewers, contact tracing, and locating personnel) have much of the field training and experience, which is necessary, and can be easily mobilized to address major public health challenges, such as a bioterror attack. Health departments need to develop plans to mobilize these types of employees for potential events. We should also assume that in a large event, hospitals and acute care providers may be overwhelmed with acute care casualties, and will be unable to provide surge capacity staffing for ambulatory care management.

Despite the 2001 experience, the literature provides little insight into planning the subacute response. Interestingly, the only paper specifically addressing this was by Gullion [11], who identified school nurses as a potential resource. Focusing on a community of 500,000 in North Texas, she calculated that to vaccinate or treat the entire population within 5 days, a minimum of 1,080 professional medical or nursing staff would be required. She also identified that hospital nurses could not be diverted, and that primary care clinics would be overrun. School nurses were identified as a resource for the subacute response, as they can be easily trained and mobilized, and have experience dealing with ambulatory populations.

4.   Lessons Learned – The Subacute Clinical Response

Preparing for local subacute response capacity is critical. Most emphasis to date has been on emergency medical services, first responders, and acute care. However, little planning has been implemented for establishing long-term follow up and capacity for providing care to subacute individuals. Civil health authorities have few direct hires on staff that can provide direct clinical service. Therefore, in the event of an emergency, most civil health authorities would have to rely on the private sector and on volunteers. Because in these environments, these services may be overwhelmed that may be difficult to rely on. Our experience and the published reports from New York and Washington clearly indicate that staff at traditional public health services were easily trained and deployed rapidly.

Initial issues, which we addressed in developing our response, were:

1. Identifying the appropriate resources, both clinical resources, personnel resources, and materials.
2. Developing appropriate protocols and algorithms. This was performed (in my mind effectively) by groups of highly trained and diverse individuals, who operated well in this type of environment.
3. Securing supplies was a major problem, especially medications. However, utilizing existing channels and providing liaison with the police in order to perform escort services was quickly established. Data collection is an initial issue, which is very important. This was addressed more effectively in the New York outbreaks (see below).
4. Communication to the public of resource availability. In an environment where stress and anxiety is a major concern, demonstrating that the health authorities are providing effective response is both essential from a community health sense, but also from a political sense, in demonstrating that government is clearly in control and is appropriately responding.

Follow-up care and surveillance is an important issue, which is frequently overlooked in planning. For example, in 2001 one of the major challenges was medication adherence. The Baltimore program did not have an adherence or systematic adverse event monitoring program. The published experience in 2001 from New York, Washington, and Florida estimated similar levels of adherence.

In the reported literature, over 15,000 people were treated and adherence was documented in all the sites [4, 6, 12]. In Florida, adherence was 31%, in New Jersey 61%, in the Senate Building 58%, in the Washington DC postal workers 64%, in New York City 21%, and in Connecticut 22%. Overall, approximately 44% of individuals fully completed the course of 60 days of ciprofloxacin. Approximately 42% had intermediate adherence, which was most widely defined as having missed doses within the past 24 hours to a week. Finally, one-fifth of the individuals stopped therapy prior to recommended completion date. The major reasons varied by the city and site of exposure, but included (in order of frequency) for stopping including adverse advents, concern of the long-term side effects, a low perceived risk of anthrax, and concern over the development of antibiotic resistance and that impact on their personal health at a later period of time.

Of those who stopped therapy, 24% indicated that they were saving the antibiotics for future use. This is particularly relevant in an environment where drug acquisition costs are high, and where access to antimicrobial therapy may not be as easy as one would hope. There is also concern (expressed by this author and others), that antibiotics were being diverted to a secondary market, where they can be potentially sold.

5.   Adverse Events

The ciprofloxacin adverse events frequency advent effects reported in 2001 was similar to that reported in the literature. Allergic (analphylactoid for ciprofloxacin) reactions were reported with a frequency of less than one per thousand. The most frequently reported minor adverse events were fatigue, nausea and vomiting, headache, loss of libido, yeast vaginitis infections in women, and occasional confusion with stress or depressive symptoms. No tendonitis was reported.

One of the problems in analyzing the adverse event data is the absence of control groups – either individuals exposed, who declined treatment, or a comparable group of the unexposed general population during this period of time.

Qualitative research performed by CDC authors [4] and an independent researcher [13] indicated that adherence to the long ciprofloxacin regimen was positively affected by public health interventions, especially at the postal service, where repeated visits by the public health staff to the workplace were helpful. These were opportunities, which we used to ask about adverse advents, and also demonstrated that the health authorities had concern over the workers. This type of follow-up activity was associated with increased compliance with medication. However, also of quite substantial interest, was that individuals had very poor or little recall of the information that was provided at the initial encounter. Workers also were adversely affected by the poor communication and mixed messages provided by different authorities, which in turn led to decreased trust and credibility. Therefore, information sheets and information sessions are all actually lost during the initial encounter presumably because of the stress of the initial event.

North evaluated Senate office building workers in focus groups and qualitative interviews 3 months after the attacks [14]. Workers noted that "communications were inconsistent" over time and across different authorities. This included both the internal communications and the public media outlet information. Recommendations include attempting to keep risk communication and system management consistent. No information was provided in this paper regarding clinical assessment and compliance.

6.   Lessons Learned

- The subacute response is a critical aspect of responding to a bioterrorism event.
- The subacute response frame work needs to be integrated into a fragmented health-care system, which is poorly equipped to deal with large-scale public health emergencies.
- Subacute clinical resource requires rapid development of clinical protocols and deployment of appropriate and trained personnel.
- Planning for logistical, organizational, and administrative support is required.
- Traditional public health clinical service organizations and personnel resources are an overlooked resource, and often have the training and institutional culture to provide response capacity.
- Adherence is a major problem, and strategies should be developed in order to approve adherence especially among groups, which are highly under stress.
- Clinical follow-up algorithms need to be developed and supported.
- Communication messages should include adherence messages, as well as potential information about side effects and what represents important and unimportant side effects.

References

1. General Accounting Office. Bioterrorism. Public health response to anthrax incidents of 2001. Washington, DC: United States General Accounting Office, 2003. Report No. GAO-04-152.
2. Gursky E, Inglesby TV, O'Toole T. Anthrax 2001: observations on the medical and public health response. Biosecur Bioterror 2003; 1(2):97–110.

3. McHugh M, Staiti AB, Felland LE. How prepared are Americans for public health emergencies? Twelve communities weigh in. Health Aff (Millwood) 2004 May–June; 23(3):201–209.

4. Shepard CW, Soriano-Gabarro M, Zell ER, Hayslett J, Lukacs S, Goldstein S, Factor S, Jones J, Ridzon R, Williams I, Rosenstein N. CDC adverse events working group. Antimicrobial postexposure prophylaxis for anthrax: adverse events and adherence. Emerg Infect Dis 2002 Oct; 8(10):1124–1132.

5. Blank S, Moskin LC, Zucker JR. An ounce of prevention is a ton of work: mass antibiotic prophylaxis for anthrax, New York City, 2001. Emerg Infect Dis 2003 June; 9(6):615–622.

6. Jefferds MD, Laserson K, Fry AM, Roy S, Hayslett J, Grummer-Strawn L, Kettel-Khan L, Schuchat A. Centers for Disease Control and Prevention Anthrax Adherence Team. Adherence to antimicrobial inhalational anthrax prophylaxis among postal workers, Washington, DC, 2001. Emerg Infect Dis 2002 Oct; 8(10):1138–1144.

7. Layton MC. Interview with Marcelle C. Layton, MD Assistant Commissioner, Bureau of Communicable Disease, New York City Department of Health and Mental Hygiene. Interview by Madeline Drexler. Biosecur Bioterror 2004; 2(4):245–250.

8. Partridge R, Alexander J, Lawrence T, Suner S. Medical counterbioterrorism: the response to provide anthrax prophylaxis to New York City US postal service employees. Ann Emerg Med 2003 April; 41(4):441–446.

9. Brookmeyer R, Johnson E, Bollinger R. Modeling the optimum duration of antibiotic prophylaxis in an anthrax outbreak. Proc Natl Acad Sci USA 2003 Aug 19; 100(17):10129–10132.

10. Inglesby TV, Henderson DA, Bartlett JG, Ascher MS, Eitzen E, Friedlander AM, Hauer J, McDade J, Osterholm MT, O'Toole T, Parker G, Perl TM, Russell PK, Tonat K. Anthrax as a biological weapon: medical and public health management. Working group on civilian biodefense. JAMA 1999 May 12; 281(18):1735–1745.

11. Gullion JS. School nurses as volunteers in a bioterrorism event. Biosecur Bioterror 2004; 2(2):112–117.

12. Williams JL, Noviello SS, Griffith KS, Wurtzel H, Hamborsky J, Perz JF, Williams IT, Hadler JL, Swerdlow DL, Ridzon R. Anthrax postexposure prophylaxis in postal workers, Connecticut, 2001. Emerg Infect Dis 2002 Oct; 8(10):1133–1137.

13. Quinn SC, Thomas T, McAllister C. Postal workers' perspectives on communication during the anthrax attack. Biosecur Bioterror. 2005; 3(3): 207–215.

14. North CS, Pollio DE, Pfefferbaum B, Megivern D, Vythilingam M, Westerhaus ET, Martin GJ, Hong BA. Concerns of Capitol Hill staff workers after bioterrorism: focus group discussions of authorities' response. J Nerv Ment Dis 2005 Aug; 193(8):523–527.

DETECTING AND RESPONDING TO BIOTERRORISM

Janet Martha Blatny

Forsvarets forskningsinstitutt (FFI), Norwegian Defence Research Establishment, P.O. Box 25, N-2027 Kjeller, Norway

1.   Abstract

Biological threat agents are infectious microorganisms such as bacteria, rickettsiae, fungi, viruses, or toxins with the intent to incapacitate or kill man, or to destroy livestock, crops, or food. The use of biological threat agents in biological warfare has a long history, but the recent use of anthrax spores in bioterrorism has urged the need for responding to such threats. The design of efficient and reliable detection and identification systems is a part of bioterrorism preparedness and response. Classical microbiology, immunoassays, and nucleic acid-based methods including molecular forensics are laboratory approaches for detecting and identifying various biological threat agents. These are supplementary methods needed for verification. However, the analysis results depend on the sample collection and handling. This chapter briefly summarizes some biological warfare and bioterrorism events, the threat posed by bioterrorism. Also, various methods and systems suitable for detection and identification of biological threat agents, with emphasis on environmental samples, are described.

2.   Introduction

Biological warfare is the deliberate dispersion of infectious microorganisms (i.e., bacteria, rickettsiae, fungi, and viruses) or toxins with the intent to incapacitate or kill man, or to destroy livestock, crops or food. Toxins may be produced naturally by microorganisms, plants, or animals, or even synthesized chemically. Biological weapons (BWs) are weapons containing infectious biological material and are regarded as weapons of mass destruction (WMD), or more appropriately as weapons of mass casualty [reviewed in 1, 2]. A BW is more than the biological agent alone and implies a delivery system such as a physical weapon (i.e., standard munitions,

M.S. Green et al. (eds.), Risk Assessment and Risk Communication Strategies in Bioterrorism Preparedness, 77–92.

missiles, vehicle, and artillery shell). The Biological and Toxin Weapon Convention (BTWC) that entered into force in 1975 prohibits the development, production, and stockpiling of BWs. The use of such weapons is banned under the Geneva Protocol 1925. Still, it is strongly believed that some terrorist organizations and certain states, which are parties to the Convention, do possess BW programs. It is generally believed that biological threat agents are easily acquired and that their production is by "dual-use" equipment. For civilian purposes such equipment is used for production of beer, yoghurt, vaccines, and antibiotics. There are several barriers in obtaining an effective BW, and two of the major challenges are (i) the development of a sufficiently virulent and infectious strain for the seed stock and (ii) the selection of the most appropriate dissemination method of the biological threat agent.

The Centers for Disease Control and Prevention (CDC) has established a list of biological agents and toxins that may pose a severe threat to public health and safety (http://www.cdc.gov/od/sap). The requirements for including the agent or toxin to this "select agent list" are based on the effect on human health of exposure, the degree of contagiousness, the availability and effectiveness of medical treatment, and the vulnerability of various populations. Since October 2005, the reconstructed 1918 pandemic influenza virus has been added to this list. Table 1 provides examples of potential biological threat agents. The Australia Group has provided guidelines and control lists for national export of equipment, technology, and biological material that could contribute to BW activities (http://www.australiagroup.net/).

TABLE 1. Potential biological threat agents

Microorganism	Disease	Mortality untreated	Infective dose[a]	Incubation time[d]
Bacillus anthracis	Anthrax	High	8,000–5,000 spores	1–6 d
Yersinia pestis	Plague[c]	High	100–500 cfu	2–3 d
Francisella tularensis	Tularemia	Low	10–50 cfu	2–10 d
Variola major	Smallpox[c]	High	10–100 pfu	7–17 d
Clostridium botulinum[b]	Botulinum	High	0.003 µg/kg (LD_{50})	1–5 d
Filovirus (e.g., Ebola, Marburg)	Viral hemorrhagic fevers[c]	High	1–10 pfu	4–21 d

Coxiella burnetii	Q fever	Low	30–3,000 cfu	10–40 d
Brucella spp.	Brucellosis	Low	10–100 cfu	5–60 d
Vibrio cholerae	Cholera	Low	10^3–10^6 cfu	4 h–5 d
Shigella spp.	Shigellosis[c]	Low	10–100 cfu	1–7 d
Salmonella spp.	Salmonellosis	Low	10–100 cfu	1–7 d
Escherichia coli O157:H7	STEC	Low	$<10^3$	10 h–3 d
Ricin toxin		High	3–5 µg/kg (LD_{50})	18–24 h

[a] Infective dose as aerosol [3], except for food and water pathogens [4].
[b] The toxin is the biological threat agent.
[c] Contagious human to human.
[d] d, days; h, hours.

3. Biological Warfare and Bioterrorism Events

The use of biological agents in warfare has a long history [reviewed in 1]. During the Middle Age (14th century) the Tartars catapulted bodies of plague victims over the walls of Kaffa in an attempt to initiate an epidemic upon the residents. During the French and Indian Wars (17th century) blankets containing pus or dried scabs from patients infected with smallpox were given to the Native American tribes in order to transfer the disease. The Germans used biological agents for sabotage during the First World War such as infecting animal feed and horses intended for export. The Japan's biological warfare program during the Second World War included experiments using plague, cholera, and plague on prisoners, where more than 10,000 died (Unit 731). President Nixon terminated the US offensive BW programs in 1970 after signing the National Security Decisions 35 and 44. The BW program of the Sovjetunionen still continued (Biopreparat) after signing the BTWC in 1972. In 1979, anthrax spores were accidentally released from one of the BW research facilities in Sverdlovsk resulting in 66 deaths [5]. This unintentional release of anthrax spores demonstrated the effectiveness of infection by inhalation. In 1978, KGB assassinated the Bulgarian writer and journalist Markov by stabbing him with the tip of an umbrella containing a small pellet of ricin. The Rajneeshee Cult deliberately released *Salmonella typhimurium* at salad bars and supermarkets in Oregon, USA, in 1984, causing an outbreak of salmonellosis where 751 people fell ill [6]. The dissemination of anthrax spores by letters and the postal processing and distribution centers in the United States, in 2001, resulted in 22 cases of anthrax in which five of the inhalation cases were fatal [7]. A study performed by the Swedish Defence Research Agency [8] showed that the majority of incidents between 1960 and 1999 using biological material in order to kill, incapacitate, or threaten, included frequent use of ricin, HIV-infected blood, and food contaminants (e.g., *Salmonella* spp. and *Shigella* spp.).

4.   Bioterrorism Threat

In order to assess a bioterrorism threat several factors need to be taken into account; the capability (technology and skills) and intention of the attackers, the vulnerability and the value of the action, and the harm of the biological agent [9]. There is a strong focus on the use of anthrax as a BW. This is due to the great stability of the anthrax spores (> 80 years), the effectiveness as an infectious agent by inhalation, and the easy dissemination of the spores. Many experts believe that biological threat agents may be more useful for obtaining panic and anxiety causing serious psychological impact instead of resulting in high numbers of casualties. The US senator Bill Frist stated at the World Economic Forum, Davos, January 2005 that "The greatest existential threat we have in the world today is biological" and that such an attack would occur at some time in the next 10 years. The Canadian Press reported in March 2005 that the military's intelligence arm has warned the federal government that avian flu may be a suitable biological threat agent. The 1918 pandemic influenza virus has recently been reconstructed by retrieving gene sequences from victims buried in the permafrost of Alaska and from preserved tissue samples [10, 11]. The 1918 flu virus killed approximately 40 million people and might be regarded as one of the most effective bioweapon known. Newly emerging (e.g., SARS, Hendra, Nipah, and avian flu) and re-emerging (e.g., West Nile, human monkeypox, multidrug-resistant *Mycobacterium tuberculosis*) pathogenic microorganisms are of global concern urging the needs for national preparedness plans, and the development and production of vaccines, antivirals, and other therapeutics. These infectious agents could potentially be used in a deliberate biological attack. Three accidental escapes of the SARS virus from laboratories in Singapore and Beijing were reported in 2003 and 2004 [12]. Gene sequences may be purchased from various genes synthesis firms by e-mail requests. Few companies check and compare the ordered sequences against sequences from biological threat agents and there are no national regulations requiring these firms to do so. Thus, there is a concern that terrorists may order specific virulence genes and perform genetic engineering to create new or altered pathogenic microorganisms [13].

5.   Responding to Bioterrorism

To minimize the effects of a biological attack, public health authorities need to be aware of the threat biological agents may have in biological warfare and bioterrorism.

Physicians need to be alerted and well-trained, have a high suspicion for these agents, and must recognize the clinical symptoms derived from such an infection. Symptoms of those exposed to such agents may be nonspecific and resemble common flu-like diseases. Many biological threat agents are zoonotic. Animals may show the first symptoms of a clinical infectious disease after a deliberate release of a biological agent. In such cases, veterinarians may be the first to encounter the disease caused by a zoonotic threat agent.

Planning for necessary actions, national and global coordination, responsibility, enhanced law enforcement, medical countermeasures, and implementing efficient syndromic surveillance systems are all essential parts of bioterrorism preparedness. In addition, designing efficient detection systems for early warning, and rapid and reliable diagnostic systems contributes to improve the response efforts. The avian flu outbreak in several Asian countries killing approximately 50 million chickens has revealed the need for establishing rapid molecular diagnostics for mass screening of the flu carriers to improve public health responses [14]. Early detection to a release of biological agents may decrease the infectious rate and the people exposed (Figure 1). By the time the clinical symptoms have emerged, it might be too late for treatment. In some cases, antibiotics may be effective as postexposure prophylaxis, but this treatment needs to start before the onset of symptoms.

6.   Biological Detection and Identification

Biological threat agents may be difficult to detect and identify quickly and reliable both from a civilian (public health) and a military point of view. There is a distinction between the terms "detection" and "identification". The establishment of the presence or absence of a biological agent is termed

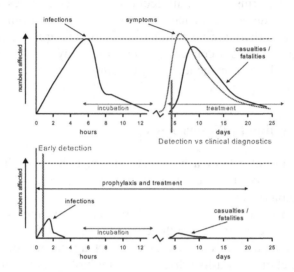

Figure 1. Early detection of a biological threat agent may reduce the number of infected individuals and casualties, and may be able to provide medical treatment before onset of symptoms.

detection, while identification is the determination of the precise nature of the biological agent. Many systems can only detect, and not identify the biological agent. The identification system is usually dependent on specific signatures (DNA, protein) of the microorganism. Identification of *S. typhimurium* as the causing strain for the deliberate outbreak of salmonellosis by the Rajneeshee Cult took 4 days, but it took more than a year to identify and confirm that only a single strain of *S. typhimurium* had been used (in addition to the confession by one of the cult members about the deliberate release). This illustrates that, in some cases, identification may be time-consuming. Many bacterial threat agents occur naturally, and some may be closely related to other bacteria found in the environment. Thus, it is necessary to distinguish between terrorist events, naturally occurring outbreaks, and background levels. False positives (i.e., alarm, but no agent) may arise when the biological detector device responds to detect and identify an interfering substance in the sample (contamination), which is not the actual biological agent. If a biological agent exists, but below an instrument's threshold value for detection and identification, a false negative may occur. Thus, the detection and identification schemes need to be carefully designed.

7.   Detection Systems for Biological Threat Agents

Efficient and reliable biodetection depends on the selectivity and sensitivity of the assay and system, as well as the collection and handling of the sample. A biological point detector for environmental (air) monitoring contains several components (Figure 2). A trigger may determine in real time any change in the biological background in air and discriminate between a biological threat agent and other particles in air, i.e., nonspecific detection. Particle sizers may be used as a trigger, exemplified by the Model 3321 Aerodynamic Particle Sizer from TSI and the Fluorescence Aerodynamic Particle Sizer FLAPS2 from Defence R&D Canada. The FLAPS2 measures the intrinsic fluorescence produced by living microorganisms. Using an ultraviolet (UV) laser, the wavelength 266 nm excites fluorescence from the amino acids tryptophan and tyrosine, while 355 nm excites fluorescence from the cofactor NADH. A stand-off detector, such as light detection and ranging (LIDAR) may also be used as a trigger and for detecting potential biological threat clouds. LIDAR is regarded as a *detect-to-warn* system [15]. Short-range LIDARs can detect at a radius of approximately 5 km from the instrument. Most LIDARs use UV radiation at 266 nm or 355 nm such that biological material will fluoresce, but UV excitation may also fluoresce fuel oils, diesel, and agrochemicals causing false alarms. So far, LIDAR is not sufficiently operative during full daylight and needs good environmental conditions to function efficiently.

A collector is used for concentrating the biological particles in air usually into a liquid. Spores, bacteria, and viruses are usually together or attached to dust and other particles in air. Thus, the term "agent-containing particles per liter of air" (ACPLA) has been adopted. The first step in detecting ACPLA is to collect large enough air samples through a collector. The impinger SpinCon® air sampler from Sceptor Industries collects particles at a flow rate of 450 l/min in the range of 0.2–10 μm into a liquid. OMNI 3000, based on the SpinCon® technology, and the Biotrace Intelligent Cyclone Air Sampler (ICAS) collects air with a flow rate of 300 and 750 L/min, respectively. The BioCapture 650 from MesoSystems is a portable handheld air collector, suitable for first responders, sampling at a flow rate of 200 L/min. The efficiency of air collection is also dependent on the size of the particles. FFI is using both the SpinCon® and OMNI 3000 air collector for outdoor and indoor sampling of air (Figure 3). These air samples are spiked with biological threat agents for polymerase chain reaction (PCR) analyses and determination of the detection limit (unpublished results). In many biodetection devices the trigger and detector have overlapping or the same functions. A detector is used to determine and characterize to a certain extent the biological origin of the aerosols. Even

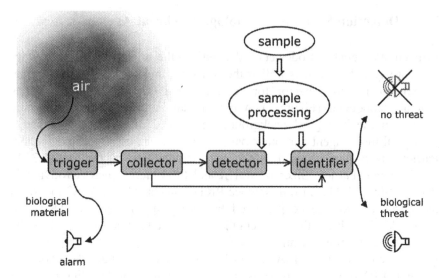

Figure 2. A biological point detection system for environmental monitoring (air) usually consists of a trigger, collector, detector, and identifier. Reliable and efficient detection and identification is dependent on the type of sample, sample collection, and sample processing.

though biological agents are detected, further identification of the agent is usually needed. An identifier performs specific identification of the biological threat agent (described in Section 5.1.8).

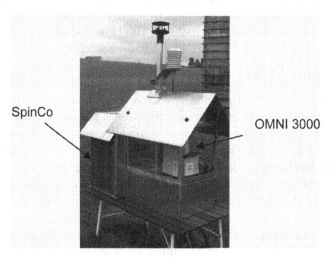

Figure 3. The SpinCon® and OMNI 3000 collector (Sceptor Industries) located outside FFI, Kjeller, for air sampling.

Biological threat agents may be present as vegetative cells, spores, or in a dormant state (viable but nonculturable state; VBNC) in environmental samples (such as water, air, and soil). ATP is frequently used for nonspecific detection of viable bacterial cells (bioluminescence assays). Some of these assays have been further improved to separate bacterial ATP from nonbacterial ATP (yeast, somatic, or free ATP), and to detect spores. Spores are deficient in ATP and a germination step is required before performing the bioluminescence assay [16, 17]. The bioluminescence assay combined with specific phage-associated lytic enzymes may be used for further identification of the bacteria.

8.   Identification of Biological Threat Agents

There are several methods available for identifying biological threat agents, but there is no single approach for identification. Definitive identification requires several methods; conventional culture-based methods immunoassays, and nucleic acid-based methods (reviewed in [18–21]), as well as clinical diagnosis of those exposed to such agents. The cultivation of bacteria in selective growth medium allows detection of viable cells, inspection of colony morphology, and determination of antibiotic sensitivity. Such classical microbiology may identify the bacterial agent at the genus level and to a certain extent at the species level. However, these methods do not identify toxins, they are time-consuming, and not suitable for first responders.

8.1.   IMMUNOLOGICAL METHODS

Immunoassays include the use of specific antibodies targeted against a toxin or a particular antigen at the surface of a bacterial cell or spore. Immunological methods usually provide quick results and are suitable for fast screening of a large number of samples. However, the method is less specific and sensitive, and the detection limit may be a 100–1,000-fold higher than the infective dose [20, 22]. In general, immunoassays are good for presumptive detection but confirmatory analysis is needed, usually by nucleic acid-based detection methods. Antibody specificity and affinity are often the limiting factors of immunoassays. Tetracore's BioThreat Alert Test strips are reagent strips using a lateral flow immunochromatography technique allowing biological threat agents to be identified within 15 min. Examples of commercially available immunological devices are the BioVeris detection system, Meso Scale Discovery Sector PR, and Luminex 100.

8.2. NUCLEIC ACID-BASED METHODS

Real-time PCR is the most commonly used nucleic acid-based method for specific and sensitive identification of biological threat agents. PCR may detect as low as 10–100 cells, but this method usually requires a clean sample. Disruption of bacterial cells and spores is often needed in order to make the DNA available for amplification in the PCR assay. An effective sample preparation may also reduce the presence of false negatives since impurities from the sample may inhibit the PCR assay. Specific identification by PCR is obtained by using specific primers and probe combinations. Each probe (e.g., TaqMan probes, fluorescence resonance energy transfer [FRET]-prober, and molecular beacons) has a different method of separating the fluorophore from the quencher when reporting the amplification process. Different reporter dyes (fluorophores) may be attached to the probes allowing simultaneous identification of several biological threat agents (multiplex identification). The PCR assay should include internal controls to avoid false positive signals. Internal controls may consist of either a plasmid or a DNA fragment in which the amplified DNA sequence is unique in the assay [23, 24].

Several real-time PCR assays have been outlined for a number of biological threat agents, and commercial kits containing the specific reagents are available. The target genes and regions for PCR identification are specifically chosen for each microorganism. For *Bacillus anthracis*, several genetic targets located on the chromosome are used for identification [25–27] in addition to the well-known target *lef*, *cya*, *pga* toxin, and *cap* capsule genes located on the virulence pXO1 and pXO2 plasmids, respectively. However, plasmid-free *B. anthracis* cells will only be identified by PCR when using specific chromosomal targets. The closest relative of *B. anthracis* is the opportunistic human pathogen *B. cereus* (soil bacterium) and the insect pathogen *B. thuringiensis*. These are functionally different, mainly distinguish by plasmid-encoded genes. The genomes of *B. anthracis*, *B. cereus*, and *B. thuringiensis* strains show a close similarity [28] complicating the search for unique chromosomal targets for thier differentiation and identification. However, genome sequencing of many biological threat agents has provided significant data about unique regions that may be suitable as specific targets for PCR identification [29]. FFI has identified one unique chromosomal target for specific identification of *B. anthracis* (unpublished results). Several real-time PCR assays for identification of various biological threat agents listed in Table 1 have been established at FFI (exemplified in Figure 4) using either the SmartCycler from Cepheid and the LightCycler from Roche Applied

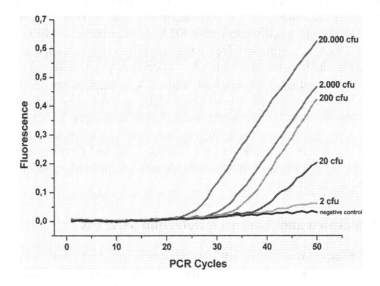

Figure 4. Identification of *Coxiella burnetti* (9 Mile, phase I) by PCR (Lightcycler™) using specific primers and probes (19).

Science (Figure 5). Idaho Technologies and Smiths detection (Bio-Seeq) have developed handheld PCR devices suitable for military use and first responders, such as Ruggedized advanced pathogen identification device (RAPID), and RAZOR, and Bio-Seeq, respectively. Bruker Daltonik GmbH has constructed a microarray system based on PCR for bioidentification. For review of various nucleic acid detection assays and systems see [18, 19, 21].

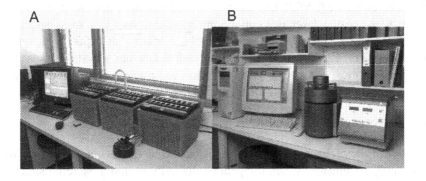

Figure 5. Real-time PCR devices at FFI. A, Smartcycler[R] (Cepheid); B, Lightcycler ™ (Roche Applied Science).

PCR can detect DNA from both viable and dead cells, and thus, culture-based methods are needed for the assessment of bacterial viability. Nucleic acid sequence-based amplification (NASBA) is a method in which RNA instead of DNA is amplified (reviewed in [30–32]). NASBA can be used to detect viable cells since mRNA is specifically detected and amplified. The design of specific primers and molecular beacons is crucial for the NASBA assay. NASBA has been widely used for virus diagnostics, and only few reports describe the use of this technique for bacterial detection. This technique has been used together with liposomal-based biosensors to identify *B. anthracis*, *Escherichia coli*, and *Cryptosporidium parvum* [33–35]. FFI has used NASBA for identification of *Vibrio cholerae* in water samples [36].

9.   Integrated and Advanced Detection Methods

Biodetection equipment for use in a battlefield is different from the use in a civilian community. If deployed in the right place and at the right time, valuable information of a bioterrorism event would be provided. The Joint Biological Point Detection System (JBPDS) is an automatic point detector for real-time identification of biological threat agents within 15 min and suitable for military use. It contains a trigger, collector, detector, and identifier, and will be used by the US Air Force and Marine Corps. Integrated systems for identification of various biological threat agents in large areas (e.g., arenas, airports) and postal service systems have been constructed, such as the Autonomous Pathogen Detection System (APDS) from Lawrence Livermore National Laboratory and the BioHazard Detection System (BDS) from Northrop Grumman, respectively.

Other biodetection techniques in advance are light scattering surface plasmon resonance (LSSPR), surface–enhanced Raman spectroscopy (SERS), and matrix-assisted laser desorption/ionization time-of-flight mass spectroscopy (MALDI-TOF-MS). There have been many attempts to develop biosensors based on electrochemics, micro-fluidics, nanocrystals (quantum dots), and optics, combined with immuno- and nucleic acid-based assays, but only few are commercially available (reviewed in [37, 21]).

10.   Molecular Forensics

Classification of bacterial strains is often based on the identification of DNA polymorphisms. When the genetic diversity within a bacterial species is high, it is often adequate to sequence only a few number of DNA fragments in order to classify the strain. In contrast, strains belonging to more homogenous species, in which little sequence divergence has occurred, it is necessary to sequence long DNA regions or to analyze several loci with high mutation rates. Variable number of tandem repeats (VNTR) is a linear arrangement of multiple copies of short repeated DNA sequences that vary in length and are highly polymorphic [38]. The size of the DNA fragments containing VNTRs is measured by PCR. Most bacterial genomes contain several VNTRs, and multi-locus VNTR (MLVA) analysis is now a suitable tool for strain typing and for tracing back to the origin of the bacterial agent [39]. VNTR analysis was used to identify the *B. anthracis* Ames strain used in the anthrax attacks in the United States in 2001 [40, 41, 29]. The United States has recently established a laboratory known as the National Bioforensics Analysis Center (NBFAC) operating together with the Federal Bureau of Investigation (FBI) [42]. The laboratory will handle an end-to-end analysis from sample collection to molecular typing. MLVA techniques have already been established at FFI and are used for genetic fingerprinting of *B. cereus* and *V. cholerae strains* (unpublished results).

11. Conclusion

Biological threat agents for the use in biological warfare or bioterrorism are infectious microorganisms or toxins with the intent to incapacitate or kill man, or to destroy livestock, crops, or food. An essential part of bioterrorism preparedness and response includes the design of efficient and reliable systems for detection and identification of biological threat agents. Various biodetection systems for environmental monitoring are available. Many of these systems have been primarily constructed for military use. There is no single approach for identification of biological threat agents, and several methods are needed for verification. Classical microbiology, immunoassays, and nucleic acid-based methods, including molecular forensics, are laboratory approaches for detecting, identifying, and verifying various biological threat agents.

References

1. Atlas RM. Bioterrorism: from threat to reality. Annu Rev Microbiol 2002; 56:167–185.
2. Davis RG. The ABCs of bioterrorism for veterinarians, focusing on Category A agents. Vet Med Today 2004; 224:1084–1095.

3. Kortepeter M, Christopher G, Cieslak T, Culpepper R, Darling R, Pavlin J, Rowe J, McKee Jr. K, Eitzen Jr. E. USAMRIID'S Medical management of biological casualties handbook, Maryland, USA, 2001.

4. Granum PE. Smittsomme sykdommer fra mat. Høyskoleforlaget, 1999.

5. Meselson M, Guillemin J, Hugh-Jones M, Langmuir A, Popova V, Shelokov A, Yampolskaya V. The Sverdlovsk anthrax outbreak of 1979. Science 1994; 266:1202–1208.

6. Török T, Tauxe R, Wise R, Livengood J, Sokolow RA. Large community outbreak of salmonellosis caused by intentional contamination of restaurant salad bars. JAMA 1997; 278:389–395.

7. Jernigan DB, Raghunathan PL, Bell BP, Brechner R, Bresnitz EA, Butler JC, Cetron M, Cohen V, Doyle T, Fischer M, Greene C, Griffith KS, Guarner J, Hadler JL, Hayslett JA, Meyer R, Petersen LR, Phillips M, Pinner R, Popovic T, Quinn CP, Reefhuis J, Reissman D, Rosenstein N, Schuchat A, Shieh W, Siegal L, Swerdlow DL, Tenover FC, Traeger M, Ward JW, Weisfuse I, Wiersma S, Yeskey K, Zaki S, Ashford DA, Perkins BA, Ostroff S, Hughes J, Fleming D, Koplan JP, Gerberding JL, The National Anthrax Epidemiologic Investigation Team. Investigation of bioterrorism-related anthrax, United States, 2001: Epidemiologic findings. Emerg Inf Dis 2002; 8:1019–1028.

8. Melin L. Terrorism och kriminalitet. FOI report 1551-864 (in Swedish), 2000.

9. Ackerman GA, Moran KS. Bioterrorism and threat assessment. The weapons of mass destruction commission, No. 22, 2004.

10. Taubenberger JK, Reid AH, Lourens RM, Wang R, Jin G, Fanning TG. Characterization of the 1918 influenza virus polymerase genes. Nature 2005; 437:889–893.

11. Tumpey TM, Basler CF, Aguilar PV, Zeng H, Solorzano A, Swayne DE, Cox NJ, Katza JM, Taubenberger JK, Palese P, Garcia-Sastre A. Characterization of the reconstructed 1918 Spanish influenza pandemic virus. Science 2005; 310:77–80.

12. Von Bubnoff A. The 1918 flu virus is resurrected. Nature 2005; 437:794–795.

13. Aldhous P. The bioweapon is in the post. New Scientist 2005; 12:8–9.

14. Fung YW, Lau L, Yu AC. The necessity of molecular diagnostics for avian flu. Nat Biotechnol 2004; 22(3):267.

15. Baxter K, Clark JM. Set lasers to...detect. NBC International, Spring 2004, pp. 26–28.

16. Trudil D, Loomis L, Pabon R, Hasan JAK, Trudil CL. Rapid ATP method for the screening and identification of bacteria in food and water samples. Biocatalysis: Fundamentals and Applications 2000; 41:27–29.

17. Fujinami Y, Kataoka M, Matsushita K, Sekiguchi H, Itoi T, Tsuge K, Seto Y. Sensitive detection of bacteria and spores using a portable bioluminescence ATP measurement assay system distinguishing from white powder materials. J Health Sci 2004; 50:126–132.

18. Iqbal SS, Mayo MW, Bruno JG, Bronk BV, Batt CA, Chambers JP. A review of molecular recognition technologies for detection of biological threat agents. Biosens Bioelectron 2000; 15:549–578.

19. Ivnitski D, O'Neil DJ, Gattuso A, Schlicht R, Calidonna M, Fisher R. Nucleic acid approaches for detection and identification of biological warfare and infectious disease agents. BioTechniques 2003; 35:862–869.

20. Peruski Jr. LF, Peruski AH. Rapid diagnostic assays in the genomic biology era: detection and identification of infectious disease and biological weapon agents. BioTechniques 2003a; 35:840–846.

21. Lim DV, Simpson JM, Kearns EA, Kramer MF. Current and developing technologies for monitoring agents of bioterrorism and biowarfare. Clin Microbiol Rev 2005; 18:583–607.

22. Peruski AH, Peruski Jr. LF. Immunological methods for detection and identification of infectious disease and biological warfare agents. Clin Diagn Lab Immun 2003b; 10:506–513.

23. Charrel RN, la Scola B, Raoult D. Multi-pathogens sequence containing plasmids as positive controls for universal detection of potential agents of bioterrorism. BMC Microbiol 2004; 4:1–11.

24. Inoue S, Noguchi A, Tanabayashi K, Yamada A. Preparation of a positive control DNA for molecular diagnosis of *Bacillus anthracis*. Jpn J Infect Dis 2004; 57:29–32.

25. Rastogi VK, Cheng T. Identification of anthrax-specific signature sequence from *Bacillus anthracis*. Proc. SPIE 2001; 4378:115–126. Chemical and Biological Sensing II (Gerdner, ed.).

26. Bavykin SG, Lysov YP, Zakhariev V, Kelly JJ, Jackman J, Stahl DA, Cherni, A. Use of 16S rRNA, 23S rRNA, and *gyrB* gene sequences analysis to determine phylogenetic relationships of *Bacillus cereus* group microorganisms. J Clin Microbiol 2004; 42:3711–3730.

27. Bode E, Hurtle W, Norwood D. Real-time PCR assay for a unique chromosomal sequence of *Bacillus anthracis*. J Clin Microbiol 2004; 42: 5826–5831.

28. Helgason E, Økstad OA, Caugant DA, Johansen HA, Fouet A, Mock M, Hegna I, Kolstø AB. *Bacillus anthracis, Bacillus cereus*, and *Bacillus thuringiensis* – one species on the basis of genetic evidence. Appl Environ Microbiol 2000; 66:2627–2630.

29. Fraser CM. A genomics-based approach to biodefence preparedness. Nat Rev 2004; 5:23–33.

30. Chan AB, Fox JD. NASBA and other transcription-based amplification methods for research and diagnostic microbiology. Rev Med Microbiol 1999; 10:185–196.

31. Deiman B, van Aarle P, Sillekens P. Characteristics and applications of nucleic acid sequence-based amplification (NASBA). Mol Biotechnol 2002; 20:163–179.

32. Cook N. The use of NASBA for the detection of microbial pathogens in food and environmental samples. J Microbiol Methods 2003; 53:165–174.

33. Hartley HA, Baeumner AJ. Biosensor for the detection of a single viable *B. anthracis* spore. Anal Bioanal Chem 2003; 376:319–327.

34. Baeumner AJ, Pretz J, Fang SA. universal nucleic acid sequence biosensor with nanomolar detection limits. Anal Chem 2004a; 76:888–894.

35. Baeumner AJ, Leonard B, McElwee J, Montagna RA. A rapid biosensor for viable *B. anthracis* spores. Anal Bioanal Chem 2004b; 380:15–23.

36. Fykse EM, Skogan G, Davies W, Olsen JS, Blatny JM. Detection of viable *Vibrio cholerae* cells by NASBA. Manuscript in preparation, 2005.

37. Deisingh AK, Thompson T. Biosensors for the detection of bacteria. Can J Microbiol 2004; 50:69–77.

38. Van Belkum A, Scherer S, van Alphen L, Verbrugh H. hort-sequence DNA repeats in prokaryotic genomes. Microbiol Mol Biol Rev 1998; 62:275–293.

39. Lindstedt BA. Multiple-locus variable number tandem repeats analysis for genetic fingerprinting of pathogenic bacteria. Electrophoresis 2005; 26:2567–2582.

40. Keim P, Price LB, Klevytska AM, Smith KL, Schupp JM, Okinaka R, Jackson PJ, Hugh-Jones ME. Multiple-locus variable-number tandem repeat analysis reveals genetic relationships within *Bacillus anthracis*. J Bacteriol 2000; 182:2928–2936.

41. Read TD, Peterson SN, Tourasse N, Baillie LW, Paulson IT, Nelson KE, Tettelin H, Fouts DE, Eisen JA, Gill SR, Holtzapple EK, Økstad OA, Helgason E, Rilstone J, Wu M, Kolonay JF, Beanan MJ, Dodson RJ, Brinkac LM, Gwinn M, DeBoy RT, Madpu R, Daugherty SC, Scott Durkin A, Haft DH, Nelson WC, Peterson JD, Pop M, Khouri HM, Radune D, Benton JL, Mahamoud Y, Jiang L, Hance IR, Weidman JF, Berry KJ, Plaut RD, Wolf AM, Watkins KL, Nierman WC, Hazen A, Cline R, Redmond C, Thwaite JE, White O, Salzberg SL, Thomason B, Friedlander AM, Koehler TM, Hanna PC, Kolstø AB, Fraser CM. The genome sequence of *Bacillus anthracis* Ames and comparison to closely related bacteria. Science 2002; 296:2028–2033.

42. Budowle B, Schutzer SE, Ascher MS, Atlas RM, Burans JP, Chakraborty R, Dunn JJ, Fraser CM, Franz DR, Leighton TJ, Morse SA, Murch RS, Ravel J, Rock DL, Slezak TR, Velsko SP, Walsh AC, Walters RA. Toward a system of microbial forensics: from sample collection to interpretation of evidence. Appl Environ Microbiol 2005; 71:2209–2213.

SPECIES-NEUTRAL DISEASE SURVEILLANCE: A FOUNDATION OF RISK ASSESSMENT AND COMMUNICATION

David R. Franz
Midwest Research Institute, MD, USA Kansas State University, KS, USA and the University of Alabama at Birmingham, AL, USA

1.   Introduction

In late June 1999, an unusual number of dead birds were reported in the borough of Queens, New York City. After 6–8 weeks, an unusual number of human cases of encephalitis were first noted in hospitals in the area. The disease was soon diagnosed as St. Louis encephalitis, a mosquito-borne viral encephalitis, the causative agent of which does not kill birds. Approximately 2 weeks after the first human cases, the "St. Louis" outbreak was announced and mosquito control began. Then, 2–3 weeks later, animal disease data and human disease data were integrated, and the true causative agent, West Nile virus, was implicated in both the bird and the human deaths. We will never know if, or exactly how many, lives and dollars might have been saved by knowing 6 weeks earlier that a new, deadly zoonotic arbovirus had been introduced to North America, but experts agree days – and sometimes even hours – make a real difference when dealing with infectious outbreaks. Had we been thinking in terms of disease – wherever it occurs – rather than just human disease, we might have done better.

Two real concerns of the time in which we live are the threat of biological terrorism and the reality of naturally emerging disease. Risk assessment and communication are central to protecting lives and property before and during an outbreak of infectious disease, whether natural or intentional. Becoming aware of any disease outbreak –natural or introduced – as early as possible, should be our highest priority. Only when we know what is going on around us can we respond and break the cycle of transmission. Not all microbes have the same impact across species, but the index case may not always be a human. Although *Bacillus anthracis* is very high on the threat list for terrorist use against humans, it is not typically transmissible and is thus of little concern for livestock. On the

M.S. Green et al. (eds.), Risk Assessment and Risk Communication Strategies in Bioterrorism Preparedness, 93–99.

other hand, a number of arthropod-borne viruses, such as Rift Valley fever virus could have broad implications for both livestock and humans, and even for wildlife. Finally, we face contagious agents, such as avian influenza virus, typically a disease only of birds, which through recombination has become a lethal human pathogen. In addition to West Nile encephalitis and avian flu, other recently emerged viral diseases – severe acute respiratory syndrome (SARS) and monkey pox – occurred first in animals. Whether a disease develops naturally or is introduced by a terrorist, an integrated network of species-neutral surveillance, supported by a deep research base and systems of communication between all sectors, will give days or weeks advanced warning of an outbreak. Therefore, monitoring the space where humans, animals, and microbes meet, while requiring some special tools and strange new agency relationships, will pay huge dividends in lives and resources saved. Disease surveillance and integration of the resulting data must be closely linked to risk assessment and communication activities.

2.   Biological Security and Human Security

Biological security is fundamental to human security; human security is fundamental to stability in this ever smaller and more connected world. If we are to be as effective as we possibly can be with our risk assessment and communication, we must first understand the playing field. The perceived threats to our biological security cover a broad spectrum world wide; where each of us finds ourselves on that spectrum depends to a great extent in which part of the world we reside. Figure 1 depicts the relative importance of the components of the threat spectrum: the enormous impact of chronic diseases such as HIV/AIDS, malaria, tuberculosis, and hepatitis; the potentially very significant impact of emerging disease, such as SARS and highly-pathogenic influenza; the potentially large impact, but low likelihood of bioterrorism and the emerging concern regarding the exploittation of dual-use biotechnologies to cause harm. The arrows demonstrate regional differences in concern regarding various aspects of the threat spectrum. Therefore, threat perception is related to technological advancement, state of public health and political factors within a given region or country. Where a country or region finds itself on the spectrum will change over time with these factors as well.

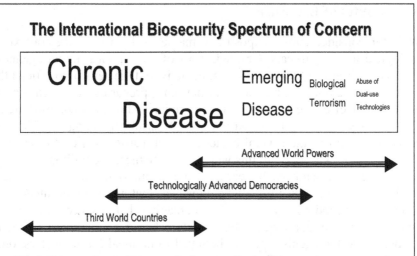

The International Biosecurity Spectrum of Concern

Chronic Disease

Emerging Disease

Biological Terrorism

Abuse of Dual-use Technologies

Advanced World Powers

Technologically Advanced Democracies

Third World Countries

Fig. 1 The spectrum of biosecurity threats. Font within spectrum represents relative health impact. Arrows depict the differing perceptions regarding type of threat in different regions of the world.

3. Natural vs. Intentional Disease

Health or economic threats to humans, animals, or both humans and animals caused by biological agents may also be categorized as natural, accidental, or intentional. Variola virus, the causative agent of smallpox, is a threat only to humans; eradicated from the globe nearly 30 years ago, it is no longer a natural threat. It could, however, be reintroduced into the human population intentionally or accidentally. *B. anthracis*, the causative agent of the disease anthrax, can affect both humans and animals. Because it is not contagious, as is variola, one would not expect there to be an accidental release of significance. There are, however, natural cases throughout the world every year and it is believed to be one of the most important agents for intentional warfare or terrorist release. The foot and mouth disease virus is the most contagious agent known to man. Although it affects only cloven-hoofed animals, it has historically, and could in the future, have an enormous negative economic impact in animal populations, which it infects. It could be introduced naturally, accidentally, or intentionally. Note that, although there are examples, such as variola and the foot and mouth disease virus, which do not cross between humans and animals, the vast majority of agents, which we might have to deal with in the future following natural, accidental, or intentional introduction affect both humans and animals.

4.   Routes of Exposure

We often consider aerosol exposure of masses of humans in the context of biological terrorist threats. Granted, most of the classical threat agents – anthrax, tularemia, Q fever, etc. must be delivered via aerosol to efficiently infect large numbers of humans. Furthermore, preparing and releasing an agent as an effective aerosol is not a trivial technical accomplishment. Disease may also be introduced via food or drink. Some agents, such as botulinum toxin or the several bacteria, which cause enteric diseases, are well suited to distribution in this way. Certainly there are millions of cases of disease worldwide each year resulting from oral exposure through food or drink. We typically believe, however, that a successful intentional attack on our food supply will be less damaging than a successful aerosol attack on one of our cities. This belief is based on both the route of exposure and the agents typically believed to be ideal for aerosol vs. oral exposure. A third mode of introduction of disease into a population might be through insect or animal vectors. The natural introduction of West Nile encephalitis virus into the United States in 1999 is an example of an agent maintained in nature and transmitted by insects; it could have been introduced by insects or birds. Although there are exceptions, most of the agents of concern from aerosol, food and drink, or vector introduction do not spread easily from person to person or animal to animal; they are not highly contagious. A fourth category of exposure modes is that illustrated by the causative agents of SARS, influenza, smallpox, and foot and mouth disease. These need only be introduced into a population. Because of their propensity to multiply in the respiratory system and/or their tropism for cells of the respiratory tract, they can spread through a population without the aid of man-made aerosols, food, or insects. Therefore, in theory, highly contagious agents need only be introduced to one or a few members of a population to cause infection and even disease in many.

5.   Discovering Disease where it Begins

In most incidences of widespread disease in a population – whether animal, human, or zoonotic – there is an index, or first, case followed by others. Depending on numerous factors, which we might simply describe as the epidemiological situation, the number of cases will first increase at some rate for a period of time and then, typically, decrease over time as well. Whether the disease is introduced naturally, accidentally, or intentionally, one of the very most important factors is discovering it as early as possible and understanding its spread through the population. Because many diseases of concern to humans are first seen in animals – West Nile encephalitis, SARS, monkey pox, H5N1 influenza are recent examples – it is critical that we seek to discover disease in the species of origin. Finding evidence of a zoonotic disease first in animals will very likely allow preventive or prophylactic actions to be taken to protect the human population. The concept of species-neutral disease surveillance acknowledges that we must look for 'disease', not 'human disease' and 'animal disease'. Finally, we live in a much smaller world than we did just a few decades ago. Transportation and travel are such that an outbreak in one part of the world today can impact humans or animals on the other side of the globe tomorrow. Therefore, there is great benefit in discovering an outbreak (1) as early as possible, (2) in the host species of origin, and (3) in the region of origin.

Traditionally, disease surveillance in most countries has involved a Ministry of Health network that monitors human disease and a Ministry of Agriculture, which monitors disease in animals. Even in the 21st century – in modern, technologically advanced democracies – it is not uncommon for these two activities to go on in parallel, sometimes discovering the same outbreak in their own species of responsibility, without effective communication between them. During the recent US introductions of West Nile virus and monkey pox, for example, communication between the animal health and human health professionals was less that adequate. Likewise, nations have been reticent to tell other nations that they have discovered a disease outbreak on their soil, fearing negative travel, trade, and economic consequences. The same attitudes and practices have been the norm in many nations and regions throughout the era of modern public health. After the hard-learned lessons described above, there is now evidence of cracks in the walls of parochialism and politics that have slowed our response to disease outbreaks for so many years at great cost in lives and wealth. Knowing that ~75% of emerging infections diseases and many of those agents traditionally selected for use as weapons are zoonotic – transmissible from animal to man – it only makes sense that we must integrate our disease surveillance efforts. The situational awareness that an integrated disease surveillance program provides must lie at the heart of modern risk assessment and communication, if we are to be prepared to minimize loss of life when disease outbreaks occur.

6.   How Can We Assure Awareness of an Outbreak?

Both the apparently increasing frequency with which we have faced newly emerging disease in recent years and the attacks experienced in the United States in 2001 have motivated a number of nations to take disease surveillance more seriously. Probably because we believe that we have been successful in developing chemical sensors – and we believe that 'bugs' and 'gas' are very similar – and because more engineers have been involved in recent defensive programs than medical and public health experts, environmental monitoring has become and remains popular. The advantage of sensors is that, if they are at the right place and the right time and designed to identify the agent which is used, they could warn us of disease-causing organisms in the air we breathe even before anyone becomes ill. These systems can be placed in the top 40–50 population-dense centers, operating around the clock, all year long, for tens of millions of dollars, or low hundreds. As currently configured, this system will likely not warn us of emerging disease outbreak. A second form of surveillance, data mining, attempts to cast a very wide net to discover, not disease, but human response to a disease outbreak: ambulance calls, over-the-counter medications purchased, emergency room visits, disease-related information sought. Although these passive programs can now be mechanized and might highlight trends and provide us enough information to help us connect the dots, the signal-to-noise problem with such systems complicates their utility. Both the concept of dispersed environmental sensors and passive data mining may be hard to justify for the many years that the threat will exist for the apparently very low-incidence bioterrorism attacks. Amazingly, we believe that the index case of inhalational anthrax was discovered by an astute clinician following the mailing of *B. anthracis*-laced letters in fall of 2001. There are a number of clinician-driven surveillance systems undergoing testing today. The greatest challenges of implementing an effective, clinician-driven system are probably (1) the difficulty we find in down-selecting to pick just the right system, (2) failure to have widespread connectivity throughout the various venues in which clinicians see patients, and (3) the time it takes from the clinicians' busy schedule to input data. There are efforts underway to deal with the first problem, by developing one higher-level integrating information system that can take inputs from numerous disparate collection systems. Finally, (4) few clinician-driven disease surveillance systems being tested today integrate human and animal disease data. As with environmental monitoring and data mining, there are trade-offs in implementing clinician-based surveillance systems. Although we will certainly discover evidence of disease wherever systems are in place, our discovery will come when there is already disease in the population. On the other hand, it may be easier to justify long-term maintenance of clinician-driven surveillance because these systems will be valuable across the entire biothreat spectrum and as preclinical diagnostics improve and find a place in the clinic, or even the home or workplace, we may be able to move ever closer to the index case and even the index exposure, the goal of environmental monitoring.

As we think about risk assessment, situational awareness, and communication regarding the biological security threat spectrum, we must address a number of questions. How much information do we really need to prepare or respond effectively? What is the requirement, and value – of these systems for "warning" and for "situational awareness"? How can we down-select from the many systems being developed? How can we make systems truly dual-use? How can we integrate international systems and information? How can we protect patient privacy? What is the appropriate balance of technical and behavioral solutions?

Exactly how to accomplish this important task is not yet clear, but its importance is unquestionable. We must watch that "spot where the animals, humans and bugs collide". Technology would allow it today; we must not let politics or borders stand in the way. Working together, across national boundaries on this, one of the most difficult and important human security issues of our time, will not only protect our citizens from natural disease, but will also build understanding and even trust that will reduce the likelihood that intentional outbreaks will be used against them.

Part II

RISK COMMUNICATION

INTRODUCTION TO BIOTERRORISM RISK COMMUNICATION

Itay Wiser[1]and Ran D. Balicer[2]

[1]*Italy Wiser, MD. Department of Epidemiology and Preventive Medicine, School of Public Health, Sackler Faculty of Medicine, Tel Aviv University*

[2]*Ran D. Balicer, MD, MPH*
Epidemiology Department, Faculty of Health Sciences, Ben-Gurion University of the Negev, Beer-Sheva, Israel

1.   Pre-event

1.1.   SHOULD WE CURRENTLY INFORM THE PUBLIC ON THE POTENTIAL RISK OF A BIOTERRORISM EVENT? IF SO, HOW?

One basic paradigm that lies at the base of many risk communication theories claim that the more we trust the people who are supposed to protect and inform us, the less afraid we will be, and the less we trust them, the greater our fears. If the public trusts the government is dealing with a crisis effectively, there will be less public fear. Still, ideal sense of partnership and trust between authorities and the public is far from present, as repeated surveys have shown. A well-planned communication effort should provide clear precautions, reassure the public, reduce unnecessary distress, and limit inappropriate demands on health-care system [1–3].

Different views exist regarding disclosing to the public preparedness plans for various scenarios of bioterrorism and as to the extent in which the public should be involved. The older paradigm claims that people should know only what the communicators want them to know, in order to get them to behave "rationally" during a crisis – i.e., the way the communicator wants them to behave [2]. This model is criticized by risk communication experts to be "overtly manipulative" and unlikely to succeed. Risk communication is more likely to succeed if it sets the more realistic goal of helping people understand the facts, in ways that are relevant to their own lives, feelings, and values, so they are empowered to put the risk in perspective and make more informed choices [4]. More updated models shift towards giving the public a sense of partnership in the emergency,

M.S. Green et al. (eds.), Risk Assessment and Risk Communication Strategies in Bioterrorism Preparedness, 103–116.
© 2007 *Springer.*

rather than conveying the minimum necessary information to keep them calm [5]. Some authors suggest that a citizen advisory panel, comprised of community members respected by and credible to their peers, can be affective mechanism for gaining constructive public participation and dialogue about possible high-concern situations [6].

Public health and media professionals generally agree that the public should be informed, and that risk communication must be tailored to fit specific scenarios, subpopulations and communication media. Still, no consensus exists on the question of how much information should the public be exposed to and what is the appropriate media for it. Furthermore, the scarcity of bioterrorist events makes it even more difficult to reach evidence-based conclusions. Therefore, risk communication experts rely mainly on behavioral theories when planning communication strategies, designing media messages, and analyzing public feedback.

Growing awareness to public communication issues has revolutionized risk communication policies. To prepare risk communication plans at the population level, models such as social amplification of risk model, may be implemented. This model is based on the theory that risk events are portrayed through various signs and images in the media, which interact with a range of psychological, social, institutional, and cultural processes that intensify or attenuate risk perceptions. This model may be helpful in analyzing the ability of agencies to work together, and it highlights the importance of incorporating feedback from the public and media to allow ongoing improvement. On that matter, recent research has established the utility of rapid polling for making informed government responses in an ongoing emergency [7].

Many of the health and risk communication theorists emphasize the need for the careful crafting of the message to be delivered, the choice of suitable and credible spokespersons, timing of message delivery, and the appropriate selection of communication channels [8, 9]. Others stress out the importance of a thorough situational analysis, consideration of the emotional and political climate, provision of information to meet the needs of the intended audience, and respect for people's capacities [10, 11].

In view of the challenges associated with heterogeneous literacy among various subpopulations, efforts should be directed at drafting messages that can reach and be understood by as many target groups as possible. This would enhance the chances that the messages will be centrally processed and achieve the best results, as outlined by the elaboration likelihood model (ELM) [12]. The ELM is based on the individual's ability to process a message and determine whether it is processed through "central" or "peripheral" route. Each route may lead to persuasive results, but the central route, which is correlated with high motivation and better message-processing mechanisms, leads to more enduring attitude and behavioral change [13]. Under circumstances of an attack, its mere threat may produce less motivation, and together with high levels of illiteracy in the American public, may be the cause of diminished ability to process complicated messages, thus leading to "peripheral route" message processing.

At the individual level, models such as McGuire's persuasion/communication model assist in increasing the likelihood of reaching an effective message by analyzing the characteristics of the input message (agency reputation, message content, and media channel) and their effect on the output (levels of persuasion and behavioral change as a result). Studies have recently shown that most local public health and health-care professionals lack adequate training and resources to carry out important communication functions. The persuasion/communication model can serve a guideline for health professional training in risk communication [5, 14].

1.2.   HOW CAN WE PREPARE NOW IN ORDER TO PERFORM BETTER RISK COMMUNICATION DURING AN EVENT?

Lessons from the anthrax mail bioterrorist attack stress out the need to prepare in advance to a bioterrorist event. Such preparedness efforts should include:

1. Ensuring collaboration and integration of agencies responsible for communication
2. Establish communication planning for bioterrorism preparedness
3. Estimate public risk perceptions
4. Prepare media information protocols in advance
5. Develop effective media-based dissemination plans
6. Design open, accurate, and consistent messages and ensure ethical approach to communication preparedness [15].

To maintain an effective risk communication policy, we should assess key elements in the public perception of risk such as familiarity of the risk, its potential damage, level of public uncertainty, public sense of control, and public trust in authorities. Legitimate sense of control can be given to those under threat, especially in advance of an attack, by public education, by public participation in the preparation process, and by providing the public a voice in the decisions that will affect them [6, 16].

The use of quantifiable scientific methods such as surveys, polls, and public interviews among various subpopulations can help identify the key risk communication messages that audiences want, need and are the most likely to be effective. A systematic communication program should begin with formal analyses identifying the core set of critical facts that impact the individuals' decision-making process, and proceed to create, evaluate, and disseminate appropriate messages. Its success could be determined with a tracking survey, assessing public mastery of those facts [2, 17, 18].

Such evidence-based data is scarce. For example, the National Institute of Mental Health's (NIMH, 2002) consensus report on early intervention after mass trauma acknowledges that the current evidence from randomized, well-controlled trials cannot definitively confirm or refute the effectiveness of such early interventions. However, even this limited evidence does permit several conclusions:

1. Any early intervention should consider the hierarchy of a victim's needs, including safety, food, and shelter.
2. The important elements of early intervention activities are an assessment of needs, the dissemination of information and the education of directly affected individuals and the general public, and the facilitation of natural support networks [19].

Rudd et al. have compared two communication efforts made by the government concerning the AIDS/HIV epidemic in 1988 and 2001 postcard sent following the anthrax letters incident. Their comparison had uncovered several important lessons:

1. Although mass mailing has a limited communication medium due to its unidirectionality, it puts critical information in the hands of a large group of people and hence is a powerful tool.
2. Over 250 studies show that health-related print materials are far exceeding the reading ability of the average adult and so health communication efforts must be tailored to the literacy skills of the intended audience.
3. The importance of pre- and post-evaluation – developers of the anthrax postcard did not have as much time to seek expert advice and field-test their mailing, and hence some of the information presented was not properly understood. Generic and disease-specific communication materials should therefore be prepared and field-tested before an event occurs.
4. During crisis events, the unexpected takes center stage and recommended steps for developing communication efforts may not be followed rigorously. However, when communication planners abandon rigor in the name of expediency, effectiveness may suffer. To avoid the need for such a choice, the public health establishment should identify critical structures and processes that it could employ to improve communications in times of crisis.

Several of these lessons were suggested years ago, but they have not been implemented into practice towards the next crisis. On 22–23 June 2001, a senior-level exercise entitled "Dark Winter" that simulated a covert smallpox attack on the United States was held. First exercise of its kind, Dark Winter was constructed to examine the challenges that senior-level policy makers would face if confronted with a bioterrorist attack that initiated outbreaks of highly contagious disease. The exercise was intended to increase awareness to the threat posed by biological weapons and to bring about actions that would improve prevention and response strategies. One of the conclusions from the simulation was that individual actions of US citizens are critical to ending the spread of contagious disease and therefore leaders must gain the trust and sustained cooperation of the American people. This conclusion, unfortunately, have been challenged unsuccessfully in the response to the 2001 anthrax attacks, when public officials failed to gain sufficient public trust and form a consistent and accurate risk communication to the public [20].

1.3. WHAT IS THE ROLE OF THE INTERNET IN RISK COMMUNICATION BEFORE AND DURING AN EVENT?

Critiques of information dissemination in response to the events of 11 September 2001, highlight new increasingly important role of the Internet as an information channel and the need for strategically coordinating what is often conflicting information. For example, one analysis recognized the importance of the Internet in providing up-to-the-minute information, but also its potential for increasing confusion and uncertainty through rapid, often-uncontrolled proliferation of information and spread of rumors. Others noted that information was coming from so many sources and transmitters, it was often more confusing and contradictory than it was helpful. Thus, it is all the more essential to plan carefully to ensure consistency of messages across channels. It is also critical to conduct research to assess how the media have covered past emergencies and to better understand norms and practices of journalists in covering emergencies [5].

A key advantage the Internet has over traditional media is that the Internet provides multiple branches of information, all accessible almost simultaneously, which the user can easily maneuver between. During the anthrax threat, the Internet also allowed for innovative communication devices such as interactive tutorials on anthrax self-care (such as "X-Plain Online" from the Patient Education Institute, 2002). Furthermore, the information provided could be customized for specific interest groups. For example, asthmatics may have had different concerns from those of the general population, just as postal workers had different needs from those of the general public during the anthrax threat.

In the 2 days after the terrorist attacks, one out of four Internet users went online in addition to monitoring television and radio reports. This suggests that the Internet may aid in assessing the credibility of information users have obtained from the traditional media [21].

The Internet also allows great scope for forward planning and dissemination of information. For example, the CDC now has detailed guidelines on anthrax management on its site, and in addition, it has published guidelines as to how individuals and agencies should act in the case of outbreaks of diseases like smallpox and typhoid [1].

Information on the Internet is available to users at any time of day, and increasingly from the home. This is especially salient given that during the height of the bioterrorist threat many people were likely afraid to travel away from home. In some cases, when a number of cities issued warnings of potential threat, people preferred to stay at home or close to home; one survey published on September 15 found that "about 9% of Americans say that in the first two days after the terror attacks they cancelled some travel plans" [21].

The Internet can serve also as a "therapeutic" medium as documented during the Gulf War. When Israeli citizens were shut in sealed rooms during the Persian Gulf War, some found the nascent Internet an essential tool in maintaining psychological stability and a way to communicate with the outside world [22].

Although the above advantages of Internet as a tool for risk communication, several challenges should be considered:

1. Internet users have no definitive way to assess web site credibility and accuracy, and thus can be mislead and misinterpret the risk level. As a result, Internet has the potential not only to help but also to harm effective risk communication policy.
2. Search engines play a key role in organizing information for the public during a bioterrorist attack. The Internet industry in cooperation with the government should develop transparent protocols for organizing key information during emergency situations so that credible and validated sites are called up first when people search for information. In addition, there is a need for more systematic regulatory oversight of web site content with the promulgation of clear industry standards, as is done in the television and radio industries.
3. Several subpopulations do not have access to the Internet. The Internet cannot therefore be regarded as an exclusive data source in times of crisis.

4. There has been limited analysis of the general impact of Internet-based health information on behavior. However, there is some evidence that health information on the Internet does affect people's management and response to health risk. The Pew Internet and American Life Project has found that 61% of those who searched online for health information – or about 43 million Americans – said that the information they found on the web improved the way they take care of themselves. In addition, 44% of those who found the health information they sought online said it affected a decision about how to treat an illness or condition and 38% said it lead them to ask a doctor new questions [21].

To summarize, the Internet can serve as an attractive risk communication tool, before and during crisis. However, Public leaders should take into account its yet limited population exposure, credibility issues, and the need for internet industry cooperation.

1.4.   HOW SHOULD WE EDUCATE THE MEDIA BEFORE AND DURING AN EVENT?

The public health community has come to recognize that the media are influential actors and determinants of health behavior and outcomes [23]. These two groups (public health community and the media) rely on each other in many ways, yet have different goals. Building Credible relationship with the press can assist authorized officials to convey public messages and guidance [5].

The role of the media is central in several risk communication theories, such as social amplification model. This model takes under consideration norms and practices of news organizations that structure how events are reported. For instance, journalists favor "legitimated" institutional sources that give a sense of authority and credibility to new reports [5]. The media needs to be monitored consistently during an emergency to ensure that information being told is accurate [24].

Following bioterrorism preparedness exercises and the September 11 attacks it has became evident that the public will turn to public health leaders for information [20]. As a result there has been growing emphasis on the need for a complete public health provider – media interface that should include pre-prepared situation specific message formats, an appointed public information officer. Another lesson learned from these experiences is that maintaining an open and proactive relationship with the press in an emergency may enhance message effectiveness by enhancing community trust [25].

Risk communication policy makers should take under consideration that journalists' attention is mostly to newsworthy information and not just information of public health importance. A recent study highlights the difficulty of getting public health messages through to news audiences when the public health crisis is embedded in a larger, complex story, as happened in the anthrax attacks that came on the heels of September 11. As a result, news media had less of a focus on the public health side of anthrax than did the CDC [26].

2.   Once an Outbreak Occurs

Effective risk communication is a serious challenge during crisis events. At such times, people have difficulty processing information and hearing, understanding, and remembering what they have been told. An environment of uncertainty and ambiguity leads many to a heightened sense of anxiety. People have a tendency to assume the worst and, as a result, their distrust of government and experts may also be heightened [27].

2.1.   GENERALLY, WE SHOULD TELL THE TRUTH SHOULD WE TELL ALL THE TRUTH? ALWAYS?

Officials may believe that they are protecting the public by withholding information regarding response plans on the theory that revealing these plans will indicate potential attackers where they can strike most effectively [28]. The attacks of 2001 have shown that determined terrorists will identify vulnerabilities that are unknown to the public. More importantly, this approach ignores the role that citizens can and should play in helping set state and local priorities [29]. Based on experience in contemporary and historic outbreaks, emphasizing the public's autonomy when implementing epidemic controls can actually help minimize the number of cases and deaths [30, 31].

The Chinese severe acute respiratory syndrome (SARS) risk communication policy serves as an example to possible damage when withholding information from the public. During the SARS crisis, Chinese officials had withheld frequent updates from the public coupled with surreptitious disease containment. As the epidemic spread across China, provincial leaders withheld information from peasants on the theory that "They just won't understand" [32]. But when peasants learned their villages might be used to quarantine outsiders who had possibly been exposed to SARS, they rioted against government preparation of quarantine centers and set up makeshift roadblocks to keep out nonresidents.

Authorities should approach members of the public as peers, as decision-makers who are interested in determining the nature of the danger and acting to reduce the chance of illness for themselves and loved ones [33]. Experience from the anthrax letters bioterrorist attacks shows that the public places more trust in updates coming from public health officials and physicians than from appointees who do not have health backgrounds [34].

Decision-makers should avoid thinking that members of the public are panicking when they are merely engaging in entirely understandable behaviors, such as seeking more information, questioning authorities, and undertaking precautionary measures (even if officials believe these are unwarranted). Rather than dismissing expressions of fear, dread, or misery, leaders should acknowledge people's sense of vulnerability and ask them to bear the risk and work together toward solutions [35].

Telling all the truth sometimes might do damage as well, especially when providing public health "good news" that are unproved or quickly refuted. An excellent example is the German and Japanese announcements of premature termination of bovine spongiform encephalopathy (BSE) crisis. In November 2000, German agriculture minister Funke declared confidently that Germany was immune from BSE. Funke essentially said to the German public, "Trust us. You're safe". One week later the first sick cow was found. Not only did this create fear of the disease, but Funke's statements damaged public trust in government, and beef sales plummeted nationwide [2]. Consider the German government's response included the resignation of Funke, and his replacement with a green party member who promised to make the Ministry of Agriculture more aware of consumers' concerns. These symbolic actions were not intended to deal with the physical risk. Rather, they recognized the peril from fear and the reality that public perceptions of mad cow disease were a very real part of the problem. This was an example of effective risk communication, with actions as well as words. Trust was restored, and despite subsequent identification of more sick cattle, within a few months beef sales had returned nearly to normal.

In a similar case, following the first case of BSE was confirmed in Japan (10 September 2001), agriculture minister Takebe foolishly promised that there would not be any others. The second sick animal was found just days later. Takebe also said that the first sick animal had not been rendered into protein and put into the cattle food supply, so the disease could not spread. Within days, the government had to admit that it was wrong and that the first animal had indeed been used to produce protein for cattle feed. The press revealed that the Japanese government had suppressed a European Union document that reported that Japan was at high risk for BSE, and also had failed to impose controls on the cattle and dairy industry to keep the disease from spreading. Takebe made his third mistake by trying to reassure the public by sacking an assistant and publicly eating beef to show that it was safe. Takebe did not resign. Although fewer sick cattle have been found in Japan than in Germany, beef sales in Japan were still off dramatically months later, much longer than it took for German beef sales to recover [2].

2.2. WILL WE BE ABLE TO CONTINUOUSLY UPDATE THE PUBLIC?

Following the 9/11 attacks, Mayor Giuliani exemplified what leaders should do when faced with uncertainty. Able to offer only a rough estimate of 9/11 casualties early on, he indicated that the final number would be "more than any of us can bear, ultimately." A question of utmost importance to the public, but one that cannot be easily answered in the initial stages of a biological attack will be: "How many sick and dying are there?" As noted earlier, leaders will face a host of other questions to which there are no quick and sure answers, such as whether an outbreak is a precursor to other attacks [29].

Through early and frequent media briefings, a leader can demonstrate a commitment to keeping the public up-to-date. This practice can also help avert an official information void that may be filled by harmful speculation or less dependable sources [29]. Steps toward effective interactions with the media include setting aside any predisposition to see the press as intruders or provocateurs, establishing positive working relationships with them prior to a crisis, developing a pragmatic communications strategy to deal with the reality of 24/7/60/60 reporting, and picking and training appropriate spokespersons. Incorporating the press in training exercises improves understanding between officials and the media of their roles and challenges in a bioterrorism response. When an event occurs, leaders often believe that they are too busy managing the response to spend time with the press and, by extension, the public. Although there is some truth in this, decision-makers should appreciate that responding to the public's concerns is not a distraction from managing the crisis, but rather is *part and parcel of* managing the crisis.

Telephone-based hotlines provide both up-to-date information to the public and public feedback tool. A telephone bank at CDC during an outbreak of Hantavirus pulmonary syndrome identified 38% of confirmed cases [36]. Computerization of the system would allow for timely transfer and analysis of complete and accurate telephone call data and perhaps provide a similar layer of passive surveillance for emerging bioterrorism events [37].

Hospital personnel, private practitioners, and emergency medical workers are understandably going to be interested in their well-being and that of their families during a health emergency. Health officials and their organizational collaborators should also ensure that these critical personnel have the information they need to reduce any unwarranted reluctance to do their jobs [29].

To summarize, providing rapid and accurate information to the public during a bioterrorist event is, therefore, critical to reducing uncertainty (US Department of Health and Human Services, 2002) and should be joined by the efforts of local, state, and federal governments to enhance surveillance for a bioterrorist attack and increase lab capacity to rapidly identify a bioterrorist agent [19].

The need for readily available health care and specially trained providers cannot be underestimated. The Gulf War syndrome controversy demonstrates how complex health issues can become after a possible CBN attack and how important it is for health-care providers to have up-to-date information. When a traumatized population cannot obtain answers to health questions from knowledgeable providers, misinformation fills the void and concerns multiply. Moreover, specially trained providers could maintain standardized medical records, which are important for scientific and medical–legal purposes [38].

Several experts emphasize the importance of local risk communication strategies to complement the information likely to be provided by national authorities. According to one expert, "We really don't understand the psychological context in which we are delivering our messages, nor whether they are really addressing the needs of the community. We need to better understand [it] so we can modify our messages and target our outreach" [19].

2.3. HOW REASSURING SHOULD WE BE?

At the very outset of a biological attack, leaders should prepare the community for conditions of uncertainty and a potentially prolonged crisis. Realistic descriptions of the tentative and evolving nature of authorities' understanding can offset public perceptions regarding an omniscient, omnipotent government on the one hand, or an utterly incompetent one on the other.

Over reassurance can lead to public mistrust, especially when the situation worsens. The anthrax letters case supplied good examples to it. You do not need to be an SRA president, Surgeon General, or risk communication guru to see problems in federal agencies' communication about anthrax during the fall of 2001. Among the examples noted by reporters:

1. *Providing inappropriately reassuring information*: Health and Human Services Secretary Tommy G. Thompson announced that initial victim Robert Stevens had probably been exposed to anthrax in the woods of North Carolina, even though scientists indicated that this was highly improbable.
2. *Downplaying uncertainty*: Federal officials initially dismissed the possibility that mail containing anthrax could be dangerous to postal employees.
3. *Delaying release of information*: CDC spokespeople voiced frustration at having little to report to the public because of the FBI's reluctance to share vital information. Similarly, while FBI officials had known about the suspicious letters sent to NBC since September 25, New York City officials were first notified of the situation by a doctor who treated one of the victims several days later [39].

Reference

1. Hobbs J, Kittler A, Fox S, Middleton B, Bates DW. Communicating health information to an alarmed public facing a threat such as a bioterrorist attack. J Health Commun 2004; 9(1):67–75.
2. Gray GM, Ropeik DP. Dealing with the dangers of fear: the role of risk communication. Health Aff (Millwood) 2002; 21(6):106–116.
3. Lofstedt RE. Risk communication: the Barseback Nuclear Plant case. Energy Policy 1996; 24(4):689–696.
4. Jasanoff S. Differences in national approaches to risk assessment and management. In: Symposium on managing the problem of industrial hazards: the international policy issues. Washington, DC: National Academy of Sciences, 1989.
5. Wray RJ, Kreuter MW, Jacobsen H, Clements B, Evans RG. Theoretical perspectives on public communication preparedness for terrorist attacks. Fam Commun Health 2004; 27(3):232–241.
6. Covello VT, Peters RG, Wojtecki JG, Hyde RC. Risk communication, the West Nile virus epidemic, and bioterrorism: responding to the communication challenges posed by the intentional or unintentional release of a pathogen in an urban setting. J Urban Health 2001; 78(2):382–391.
7. Blendon RJ, Benson JM, Desroches CM, Weldon KJ. Using opinion surveys to track the public's response to a bioterrorist attack. J Health Commun 2003; 8(Suppl 1):83–92; discussion 148–151.
8. Sandman PM. Hazard versus outrage in the public perception of risk. In: Covello V, McCallum D (eds). Effective risk communication: the role and

responsibility of government and non-government organizations. New York: Plenum Press, 1989, pp. 45–49.

9. Covello VT. Communicating risk information: a guide to environmental communication in crisis and non-crisis situations. In: Kolluru R (ed.). Environmental strategies handbook: a guide to effective policies and practices. New York: McGraw-Hill, 1998, pp. 359–373.

10. Wallack L. Two approaches to health promotion in the mass media. World Health Forum 1990; 11(2):143–154; discussion 155–164.

11. Backer TE, Rogers EM, Sopory P. Designing health communication campaigns: what works? Newbury Park, CA: Sage Publications, 1992.

12. Zarcadoolas C, Pleasant A, Greer DS. Elaborating a definition of health literacy: a commentary. J Health Commun 2003; 8(Suppl 1):119–120.

13. Petty R, Barden J, Wheeler S. The elaboration likelihood model of persuasion: health promotions that yield sustained behavioral change. In: DiClemente R, Crosby R, Kegeler M (eds). Emerging theories in health promotion practice and research: strategies for improving public health. San Francisco: Wiley, 2002, pp. 71–99.

14. Evans RG, Crutcher JM, Shadel B, Clements B, Bronze MS. Terrorism from a public health perspective. Am J Med Sci 2002; 323(6):291–298.

15. McLcan V. Partnership for public warning. A national strategy for integrated public warning policy and capability, 2003.

16. Slovic P, Fischoff B, Lichtenstein S. Facts and fears: understanding perceived risk. In: Schwing D, Albers R (eds). Societal risk assessment: how safe is safe enough? New York: Plenum Press, 1980, pp. 181–216.

17. Morgan MG. Risk communication: a mental models approach. Cambridge: Cambridge University Press, 2002.

18. Fischhoff B, Gonzalez RM, Small DA, Lerner JS. Evaluating the success of terror risk communications. Biosecur Bioterror 2003; 1(4):255–258.

19. Stein BD, Tanielian TL, Eisenman DP, Keyser DJ, Burnam MA, Pincus HA. Emotional and behavioral consequences of bioterrorism: planning a public health response. Milbank Q 2004; 82(3):413–455, table of contents.

20. O'Toole T, Mair M, Inglesby TV. Shining light on "Dark Winter". Clin Infect Dis 2002; 34(7):972–983.

21. Rainie L. Pew Internet and American Life Project Report: how Americans used the internet after the terror attack, 2002.

22. Ritchie EC, Friedman M, Watson P, Ursano R, Wessely S, Flynn B. Mass violence and early mental health intervention: a proposed application of best practice guidelines to chemical, biological, and radiological attacks. Mil Med 2004; 169(8):575–579.

23. Institute of Medicine. The Future of the Public's health in the 21st century. Washington, DC: National Academies Press, 2003.

24. Prue CE, Lackey C, Swenarski L, Gantt JM. Communication monitoring: shaping CDC's emergency risk communication efforts. J Health Commun 2003; 8(Suppl 1):35–49; discussion 148–151.

25. Bennett P. Understanding responses to risk: some basic findings. In: Bennett P, Calman K (eds). Risk communication and public health. Oxford: Oxford University Press, 1999, pp. 3–19.

26. Mebane F, Temin S, Parvanta CF. Communicating anthrax in 2001: a comparison of CDC information and print media accounts. J Health Commun 2003; 8(Suppl 1):50–82; discussion 148–151.

27. Rudd RE, Comings JP, Hyde JN. Leave no one behind: improving health and risk communication through attention to literacy. J Health Commun 2003; 8(Suppl 1):104–115.

28. Connolly C. Bioterrorism preparedness still lacking, health group concludes. Washington Post, 12 December 2003, A02.

29. Leading during bioattacks and epidemics with the public's trust and help. Biosecur Bioterror 2004; 2(1):25–40.

30. Leavitt JW. Public resistance or cooperation? A tale of smallpox in two cities. Biosecur Bioterror 2003; 1(3):185–192.

31. Annas GJ. Bioterrorism, public health, and civil liberties. N Engl J Med 2002; 346(17):1337–1342.

32. Beech H. The quarantine blues: with suspected SARS patients getting dumped in their backyards, China's villagers rebel. Time Asia Magazine, 19 May 2003.

33. Blendon RJ, Benson JM, DesRoches CM, Pollard WE, Parvanta C, Herrmann MJ. The impact of anthrax attacks on the American public. MedGenMed 2002; 4(2):1.

34. Survey shows Americans not panicking over anthrax, but starting to take steps to protect themselves against possible bioterrorist attacks. Harvard School of Public Health press release.

35. Centers for Disease Control and Prevention. Crisis and emergency risk communication. Atlanta, GA: CDC, 2002.

36. Tappero JW, Khan AS, Pinner RW, Wenger JD, Graber JM, Armstrong LR, et al. Utility of emergency, telephone-based national surveillance for Hantavirus pulmonary syndrome. Hantavirus Task Force. JAMA 1996; 275(5):398–400.

37. Mott JA, Treadwell TA, Hennessy TW, Rosenberg PA, Wolfe MI, Brown CM, et al. Call-tracking data and the public health response to bioterrorism-related anthrax. Emerg Infect Dis 2002; 8(10):1088–1092.

38. Hyams KC, Murphy FM, Wessely S. Responding to chemical, biological, or nuclear terrorism: the indirect and long-term health effects may present the greatest challenge. J Health Polit Policy Law 2002; 27(2):273–291.

39. Chess C, Celia J. Risk communication is a key to dealing effectively with bioterrorism. Risk Anal 2002; 22(6):1039–1040.

RISK COMMUNICATION TO HEALTH-CARE WORKERS AS A RISK REDUCTION MEASURE IN BIOTERRORISM

Yoav Yehezkelli, Yoram Amsalem, and Adi Aran
CBRN Medicine Branch
IDF Medical Corps

1. Abstract

A Bioterrorism act is a possibility perhaps more realistic today then ever before. Health-care workers will always be in the forefront of mitigating disease. In case the offending agent is contagious, the outbreak might spread from person to person, medical personnel being in specific jeopardy because of their increased contact with ill people. Spread among medical staff was an important route in propagation of the severe acute respiratory syndrome (SARS) epidemic in 2003. Infection control measures have proved invaluable in halting the progress of the epidemic.

Fortunately, medical personnel neither encounter highly contagious illnesses, nor bioterrorism, in their daily practice. One must therefore assume that there will be increased anxiety among health-care workers in the face of an unfamiliar disease. A bioterrorism event can be caused by a vast range of agents, which differ considerably in their contagiousness and risk to the environment. An inappropriate perception of the true risks in case of a bioterrorism event might lead to improper actions being taken either due to under estimation or over estimation of the risk. Work absenteeism might be another undesirable effect.

Understanding the real risks associated with bioterrorism events will serve both to diminish anxiety and uncertainty among health-care workers, and to allow them to take proper infection control measures, as well. These, in turn, will aid in prevention of further spread in case of a contagious agent outbreak. Instruction of the subject in peacetime, as well as preparing for appropriate risk communication in real time will serve this purpose.

M.S. Green et al. (eds.), Risk Assessment and Risk Communication Strategies in Bioterrorism
Preparedness, 117–121.

2.   Introduction

Bioterrorism is a possibility perhaps more realistic today than ever before. Although its probability is low, consequences might be vast. The product of multiplying the probability and the damage reflects the impact of an event and on how much resources should be allocated to prepare for it.

Once a bioterror (BT) agent has been released it infects those who were primarily exposed. Secondary spread occurs as a result of person to person transmission in case of a contagious disease. Health-care workers contact with ill people, being in close are at increased risk for being infected and serve, unintentionally, as a vector for further transmission. In 2003, for example, spread among medical personnel was an important route in propagation of the SARS epidemic, as was in other epidemics in history.

Diseases that are implicated as possible biowarfare (BW) agents according to the Centers for Disease Control and Prevention (CDC) lists are quite unknown to medical teams nowadays. False or inappropriate perception of the risk of their spread might lead to improper use of protective measures, both to the side of underprotection and to the side of overprotection. The most extreme protective measure health-care workers might take is not to come to work. This of course will have deleterious effects on the ability of the system to cope with a bioterrorism attack.

Fortunately, most BW agents are not contagious. Anthrax, for example, does not spread from person to person though it is highly stable in the environment, contaminates objects and even people, and might necessitate decontamination of exposed persons. Pneumonic plague and smallpox are contagious but their routes of transmission are different leading to different grades of contagiousness.

Infection control measures have been used for many years. But only in recent years their significance has been increasingly recognized, probably because of the great increase in morbidity and mortality associated with nasocomial infections. In 1996, the current guidelines for infection control in hospitals were accepted (from the CDC Hospital infection control practices Advisory Committee). These include two systems of infection control: standard precautions and transmission-based precautions.

3.   Infection Control Measures

Standard precautions are intended for all patients, regardless of their specific illness and infective state. They consist mainly of using gloves at any contact with body fluids wearing overgarments when needed, and taking care of the patient environment and disposals.

Transmission-based precautions are intended for patients infected with specific pathogens that might be transmissible. They are always being implemented as an adjunct to standard precautions. They include extra measures of PPE (personal protective equipment) targeted against the specific mode of transmission. In addition, they include requirements for specific measures for physical isolation of the patient, ranging from simple isolation in a private room to a complex total air system isolation in a negative pressure room.

The extent of implementing protective measures should fit the mode of transmission of the specific agent. There are three main transmission mechanisms:

- Contact transmission: Contact with the patient skin or from objects that have been in contact with the patient.
- Droplet transmission: Originating from respiratory secretions. These may infect in the close range (upto 1–2 meters).
- Airborne transmission: Infective droplet nuclei which might be carried by air currents for quite long distances.

Several examples of various BT agents and their mode of infectivity:

Viral hemorrhagic fevers (VHF), smallpox, glanders, and bubonic plague infect via contact.

Pneumonic plague infect by way of droplets.

Smallpox and VHF are also airborne infections. This is the most fearsome mode of transmission because airborne particles might be carried in the air for long distances and infects people that are quite remote from the ill person.

Protection from airborne infections requires placing the patient in a negative pressure room that meets international standards (Table 1). In addition, medical staff must be protected by wearing a suitable mask, verifying their vaccination status against the specific agent (when applicable) and applying other protective measures. Special consideration should be given to respiratory protection while doing some high risk procedures that carries increased risk for respiratory exposure (e.g. endotracheal intubation, bronchoscopy). In such cases it may be wise to use better respiratory protection. Table 1 summarizes the various protective levels and measures that should be implemented while taking care of patients infected with a contagious pathogen (both naturally occurring and BT agents).

Regarding airborne infections, one should remember that proper respiratory protection with N-95 standard mask is not just putting it on.

Studies have shown that unless the mask is properly fitted to the person there will be air leaks around the mask.

Therefore, it is extremely important to train health-care workers with using the protective equipment. Otherwise the protection will not be appropriate and might even give the workers a false sense of security and render them even more prone to exposure.

4.   Bioterrorism Preparedness

Infection control measures should be an integral part of every contingency plan for BW and bioterrorism. Importantly, the recommendations valid in medical facilities for routine medical care are also suitable for BT scenarios. Adherence to these guidelines on a day-to-day basis, and based on the epidemiological features of the disease, will ensure that an infectious disease will not spread, even before an outbreak is recognized as originating from BT.

Extra precautions should be implemented when specific agents are being suspected, even before the suspicion was confirmed by the laboratory.

Biohazard recommendations exist for the medical laboratories, as well. Again, their implementation on the day-to-day routine will ensure that they will be correctly used also in a BT event.

Prevention of the spread of the epidemic is a major element in BT contingency plans. As was in the SARS epidemic, it involves designating specific hospitals for the infected patients, procurement of protective equipment, special rooms, and isolation wards.

The risk from BT is real but its extent should be appropriately recognized, and appropriate perception of the risk by medical personnel will lead to appropriate protective measures being taken. Otherwise improper actions might be taken, both to the side of under-action leading to unnecessary spread and both to the side of over-action resulting in unnecessary isolations, increased anxiety among personnel, patients and relatives, and in abandonment of medical facilities by health-care workers. As most agents do not persist in the environment, usually there is no need for decontamination of patients and areas. Infectivity is usually not as high as thought. In modern times, plague is not expected to cause large-scale epidemics in developed countries, as a result of better hygienic conditions and because of the availability of effective prohylactic measures. Infection control measures in medical facilities are very important in halting the spread of epidemics, as was demonstrated in the SARS case.

Education and training is mandatory. One of the most important factors in the preparedness for a bioterrorism incident is the awareness of medical teams to the possibility of such an unusual incident. Awareness will enable early recognition of a BT incident and immediate activation of emergency plans.

5.   Conclusion

Knowledge of the real risks from bioterrorism will serve both to diminish anxiety and uncertainty among health-care workers, and will lead to implementation of proper infection control measures, as well. These, in turn, will aid in prevention of further spread in case of a contagious agent outbreak. Instruction of the subject in peacetime, as well as preparing for appropriate risk communication in real time are key elements in minimizing the impact upon the health-care system in case of a BT incident.

TABLE 1. Standard and transmission-based precautions

	Respiratory protection	Overgarments	Gloves	Patient's room
Standard	Procedures producing spray/splash	Procedures producing spray/splash	When in contact with body fluids	Regular room
Contact	Same as standard	Always	Always	Separate room
Droplet	Surgical mask	Same as standard	Same as standard	Separate room
Airborne	N95 mask	Same as standard	Same as standard	Negative pressure room

ANTHRAX-EURONET AND BEYOND – CHALLENGES OF SCIENTIFIC RESEARCH ON HIGH RISK AGENTS

Amanda J. Ozin and Stefan H.E. Kaufmann

Max Planck Institute for Infection Biology, Dept of Immunology, 21/22 Schumannstr. D-10117 Berlin, Germany

1.   Abstract

Anthrax-EuroNet and beyond: How should scientific research on potentially dangerous agents be conducted and coordinated? How should the results be disseminated to prevent the misuse of information? These questions will be addressed herein with reference to the activities and outlook of the "Anthrax-Euronet" – a research network formed to harmonize best practices in the anthrax field and to strengthen networking activities or the research community with public and private health sectors regarding preparedness to counter the threat of bioterrorism. Strategies for addressing the dual-use dilemma of research on dangerous pathogens (i.e., potential misuse of life sciences to cause harm) and the need to engage infection biology researchers in the task of improving risk assessment and risk communication approaches related to communicable diseases will be discussed.

2.   Infection Biology and 21st Century Research Priorities

2.1.   WHAT IS INFECTION BIOLOGY?

Traditionally the field of infectious disease research is bound tightly to the more clinical aspects of illness and disease. A focus on methods for rapid diagnosis and prophylactic treatments of infectious diseases teamed with public education and communication strategies have been the best defense to eliminate and/or prevent the spread of diseases. To date the number of infectious diseases outweighs the number of safe and effective vaccines, and the number of therapeutics are becoming limited by the widespread use of antibiotics and other medications, which have contributed to the rise in antimicrobial resistance in many pathogens. For the future, new diagnostic markers and novel prophylactic measures against infections are much needed to protect human and animal health. To meet these needs, the

123

M.S. Green et al. (eds.), Risk Assessment and Risk Communication Strategies in Bioterrorism Preparedness, 123–130.

relatively new field of infection biology has emerged to look more closely at the biology of host–pathogen interactions in relation to infectious diseases. Infection biology comprises scientific study of infectious agents (bacteria, fungi, parasites, viruses, and prions) and their interaction with the host at the molecular, cellular, organ, organism, and population level. It employs multidisciplinary approaches comprising concepts and methodologies of molecular genetics, immunology, cell biology, epidemiology, clinical research, and protein chemistry. With today's technology for sequencing and analysis of whole genomes (i.e., the entire genetic make-up of an organism, including humans) infection biology has taken off in new directions using a "systems" approach to look at host–pathogen interactions. This holistic approach allows one to study whole organisms and patterns of both total gene (transcriptomics) and proteins (proteomics) expression pre-, post-, and during the infection and disease process. This new paradigm in infection biology to "know our enemy and to know ourselves"[1] will surely lead us to the new knowledge, diagnostic tools, and prophylactics we need to successfully combat the threat of emerging and reemerging infectious diseases.

2.2   MAX PLANCK INSTITUTE FOR INFECTION BIOLOGY – COORDINATES ANTHRAX-EURONET

The Max Planck Institute for Infection Biology (MPIIB) was founded in 1993 as one of the first Institutes of the Max Planck Society in reunified Germany, and a special state-of-the-art research facility was erected to work with pathogens and model infection systems. The main goal of the institute was to research infectious diseases in close collaboration with universities and clinical settings. Since its short time of operation, the MPIIB has expanded rapidly in its research force and is already regarded internationally as a centre for interdisciplinary research excellence on the biology of infectious diseases at the molecular and clinical level. The institute is located in the heart of Berlin on the historical Charité medical campus, where great scientists Robert Koch, Paul Ehrlich, and Emil Behring had made their important discoveries paving the field of infection research. As one can see in the schematic map of the Charité campus, the significant positioning of the MPIIB between the Charité hospital, Berlin's renowned university hospital and medical research centre, and Germany's

---

[1] Sun Tzu [circa 400–320 B.C.] contributor to "Art of War"– translation by Lionel Giles, MA (1910). "If you know the enemy and know yourself, you need not fear the result of a hundred battles. If you know yourself but not the enemy, for every victory gained you will also suffer a defeat. If you know neither the enemy nor yourself, you will succumb in every battle."

Parliament buildings facilitates the goal of the institute to research infectious diseases in close collaboration with universities and clinical units, and also acts as a physical reminder of the role and responsibilities of the research community in both public health and policymaking.

2.3. CHANGING TIMES – NEW PRIORITIES IN MICROBIOLOGY RESEARCH

From the perspective of a microbiology researcher, "times have really changed" and research focus in the field have shifted to the small percentage of the microbial world, which actually causes diseases. Indeed, these changes are justified since facts show that infectious diseases continue to be the number one cause of death worldwide. AIDS, malaria, and TB certainly rank as the major causes of mortality and the threats of newly emerging and reemerging infectious diseases, such as SARS and possible development human pandemic influenza strain, will further compromise global public health and economy. Since the fear and panic caused by the terrorist events of 9/11 and the subsequent anthrax attacks via the US postal service pose new challenges for the 21st century through the added threat of deliberate infection by what is known as high consequence pathogens and toxins (HCPT).[2] The subsequent "biodefense funding boom" has been subject of much criticism especially when many people are dying each year of naturally occurring infectious diseases and the growing concern that funding for HCPT may be diverting much needed funds and attention from basic research in immunology and microbiology.

Other aspect of these "changing times" are the new considerations that life science researchers have to make in planning, executing, and communicating research, particularly, the question of how to strike a balance between maximizing security (i.e., biosecurity[3]) and minimizing the impacts on research to benefit public – otherwise known as the dual-use dilemma. In addition, there is growing public fear of biosafety and biocontainment issues of HCPT, especially in areas where high security and containment research facilities are being built up in their neighborhoods and with increasing media coverage of reports of accidental laboratory infections and mistakes in shipments of dangerous strains. Therefore, in

---

[2] Organisms considered to be HCPT follow the CDC proposals of classification and are subject to the US Select Agent laws – http://www.bt.cdc.gov/agent/agentlist-category.asp

[3] Biosecurity refers to ensuring the security of biological materials to prevent theft, illicit use, or release, whereas biosafety and biocontainment, denote a set of procedures and measures aimed at regulating the safe use and storage of biological materials to reduce accidental exposure or release of agents into the environment. In practical terms the concepts of security, safety, and containment are inseparable and integral to how infectious disease research should be conducted and communicated.

the context of this workshop on risk communication and risk assessment related to bioterrorism, the Anthrax-EuroNet is a model that demonstrates a "bottom-up" approach to improve research coordination and to network the research community to activities of the public health and policymaking sectors in terms of developing regulations and codes of conduct to ensure sensible biosecurity in HCPT research and communication.

3.   Security Politics, Public Health, and the Anthrax-EuroNet, Security Issues and Life Sciences Research

The use of chemical and biological toxins and organisms to cause harm is not acceptable in our modern society. The shocking use of sarin gas in the Tokyo subway system (killing 12 and injuring over 6,000) and the failed attempts to use biological weapons such as anthrax and botulism to kill people by the Japanese doomsday cult Aum-Shinrikyo-Sect (1990–1995) is a clear break of this taboo. The more recent anthrax attacks on the US postal system, demonstrates that other groups are willing to cause harm using such nonconventional weapons. In the 21st century we are faced with the challenge of increased availability of know-how and biological materials, and rapid progress in biotechnology and genetics that makes the optimization, or "weaponization," of microbial agents and toxins possible. Therefore, the potential misuse of advances in life science research for hostile purposes, or "dual-use dilemma," is a reality that requires appropriate responses from the academic, private, and public sectors. There are a number of questions that need to be addressed to help guide researchers and policymakers for 21st century life science, such as: how can we maximize biosecurity and minimize the impact on legitimate research and collaborations? How should this be regulated and the regulations implemented.

A number of significant publications propose approaches and regulations and identifies the types of high-risk research, the "Experiments of Concern,"[4] to which these guidelines should be applied. These experiments include:

1. Demonstration of how to render a vaccine ineffective
2. Confer resistance to antibiotics or antivirals
3. Enhance pathogen's virulence/render a non-pathogen virulent
4. Increase a pathogen's transmissibility

---

[4] National Research Council, Biotechnology Research in an Age of Terrorism Confronting the Dual Use Dilemma (2003): www.nap.com – Fink Committee Report

5.   Alter a pathogen's host range
6.   Enable evasion of diagnostic tests
7.   Enable weaponization of pathogens and toxins

Most seem to agree that the government should avoid implementation of regulations that would interfere with scientific progress and rather focus on supporting self-governance by scientists (i.e., self-governance vs blanket regulations). For example, trusting the scientists and publishers to screen their papers for security risks as opposed to censorship, tight regulations, and strict selection criteria for what can be published. In addition, it was suggested that research, which may fall into the above seven high-risk groups should be subject to some level of approval by the Institutional Biosafety Committees that already have the mandate to oversee recombinant DNA research at 400 US institutions. Moreover, the establishment of a National Scientific Advisory Board for Biosecurity (NSABB)[5] was recently endorsed with the mandate to provide advice to federal departments and agencies on dual use issues. Another key point is the need for international support for biosecurity. Biological information, materials, tools, and know-how are widely distributed therefore the application of national regulations, in the United States for example, would have little effect if similar measures were not encouraged globally.

3.1.   EU RESPONSES TO BIOLOGICAL AND CHEMICAL THREATS

How does the Anthrax-EuroNet project fit into the larger European Union response to the threat of bioterrorism? Post-2001 anthrax attacks, the European Union responded by initiating a broad range of actions under the auspices of Public Health and Emergency Responses.[6] The activities specific to communicable diseases focus on rapid information exchange and coordination of responses and ensure the availability of appropriate treatments. In addition, a research and development expert group was con-vened to identify means of combating biological and chemical threats. This groupconsists of national representatives from the public health and relevant academic sectors and has the mandate to:

---

[5] http://www.biosecurityboard.gov/ The first official meeting was held July 1, 2005.
[6] http://europa.eu.int/comm/health/index_en.htm

- Inventory of current research activitiesExamine how to best exploit and coordinate research
- Identify gaps and additional research needed (short- and long-term)

Most of the identified research needs have been addressed within the 6th EU Research Framework Programme (FP6) launched at the end of 2002.[7] These included projects aimed at development of fundamental knowledge and tools to counter bioterrorism (i.e., diagnostics, prevention, treatment, detection, surveillance, civil protection). In this context, the Anthrax-EuroNet project proposal addressed the gaps in knowledge related to vaccines and treatments of anthrax.

In January 2004, the Anthrax-EuroNet Coordination Action (CA), received award of funding under the Scientific Support to Policies (SSP) priority aimed at strengthening international networking activities to the public and private sectors, and to harmonize best research practices for anthrax prophylaxes development. The core consortium consists of leading European researchers and anthrax reference centres from Germany, Italy, France, and the United Kingdom. Together, these researchers focused on the difficulties that exist in comparing results of anthrax experiments performed in different laboratories, such as the many different existing animal models, strains, and protocols. Through coordinated networking activities and the establishment of standards, Anthrax-EuroNet would like to contribute to improvements in the comparability of data results for development of safer vaccines and therapeutics. Anthrax-EuroNet also hopes to become a part of larger "network of networks," which, in the future, will work to coordinate and set priorities for research into dangerous pathogens.

3.2.   SUMMARY OF ANTHRAX-EURONET CURRENT ACTIVITIES

Presently, the Anthrax-EuroNet is compiling information and performing pilot tests for drafting a handbook on *Current and Recommended protocols in Anthrax Prophylaxes Research.* These activities are based on the outcome of a questionnaire regarding key steps and source of materials in anthrax research methods. The questionnaire was distributed to leading laboratories working on these topics across the globe. Disappointingly, a number of labs had to refuse to participate in this effort because, in the absence of clear international recommendations or guidelines and, they were unsure of how "biosecurity issues" might impact on the exchange of sensitive information.[8] The consortium decided that the European participants provided

---

[7] http://fp6.cordis.lu/index.cfm?fuseaction=UserSite.FP6HomePage

[8] Ozin AJ, Bade K, Kaufmann SH. US restrictions limit anthrax networking. Nature 2004;431(7011), 883–1022.

sufficient high quality of information necessary to complete plans to compile information on protocols for anthrax vaccine and therapeutics research. Discussions of the level of dissemination of the final handbooks are underway.

Other important steps included meeting and exchanging ideas with those who could not participate in the questionnaire to find ways in the future to improve communications and exchange information (i.e., use of "Memorandums of Understanding" (MoU) until clearer regulations and ways of identifying legitimate activities have been established).

Other Anthrax-EuroNet activities include the organization of a symposium/ workshop that will convene researchers and representatives from the private and public health sectors to discuss research directions, research funding, and issues of biosecurity and scientific communication towards advancing the development of novel therapies and preventive measures to counter deliberate epidemics (Berlin, Feb. 2006). A full description of the "WHO, WHAT, and HOW" of the project and activity updates can be found at www.anthrax-euronet.com.

4.   Conclusions

There is an important triangle of risk communication related to biosecurity. The players are the public health sector, the policymakers, and the broader life sciences research community. The Anthrax-EuroNet is a project that aims to coordinate research in Europe and as well with global efforts to develop safe and effective prophylaxes for infection with *Bacillus anthracis*, by natural or deliberate release. It also functions as a forum for a "bottom-up" approach to exchange ideas and to develop protocols for sharing and communicating scientific information on anthrax and other HCPT. It is hoped that together the research community will spread a "culture of responsibility" and contribute ideas on how to deal with dual use issues and, in addition, find ways to communicate with policymakers to set the agenda for research priorities and future needs in infectious disease research. Clearly, the development of novel strategies to combat the threat of infection and for accelerating the transfer of results at the bench into viable treatments, diagnostics, and preventive measures requires funding, input from the public health sector, and political support. New concepts and some form of regulations or guidelines for exchange of scientific information and materials will be necessary for 21st-century life sciences in the context of biosecurity. Such regulations should build on already existing regulations, should address the internationality of research, and should integrate the needs of both the research community and security bodies.

Acknowledgments

I would like to thank those persons from the MPIIB who have participated in the concept, development, and administration of the project: Professor Stefan H.E. Kaufmann who is co- coordinator of the project, Dr. Robert Golinski and Dr. Karen Bade (Anthrax-Euronet office), and Birgit Arnold (Finance dept MPIIB). Moreover, I would like to acknowledge the support from the EC under the FP6 Scientific Support to Policies priority as coordinated by our former project manager Dr. Paul Vossen and currently by Dr. Arne Flåoyen. Thank you to the consortium partners and also external members consisting of researchers and our governing council.

RISK COMMUNICATION AND PUBLIC BEHAVIOR IN EMERGENCIES

Yair Amikam
Deputy Director-General for Information and International Relations,
Ministry of Health, Israel

In emergencies, the communications media have a crucial role to play in covering incidents and we have to know how to correctly exploit them. Credibility and reliability must be maintained as much as is possible within the inevitable constraints of secrecy, field security, and so on.

The media's role may be central but we must not make the mistake of inferring from that that in emergencies the media become part of the system. The media are a vital vehicle for transferring information but, even in emergencies, they will remain totally independent, capable of filtering information, voicing criticism, preferring their own sources, and so on.

Our job is to find the common ground between the establishment and the media. When any incident occurs, conventional, biological, or otherwise, the media have a crucial role to play in getting our message across to the general public; if we add that a large section of the public will be sitting at home, the media's role is second to none.

When the public is suddenly exposed to a type of incident it has not met before, any lack of information can cause hysteria, precisely because of the public ignorance of the nature of this type of incident. Communication nowadays is a 24-hour-a-day affair, constantly available in the kitchen, the car, at the workplace, and at home. Especially if people are sitting shut inside a sealed room their only channel to the outside world is the radio or television. This shows us that the communications media in Israel fill more than just a public relations or public educational function (although this role in itself is of no small importance): they are also needed for getting messages, instruction, and guidance to the public.

The establishment can make use of the media in a number of ways and for a number of purposes:

1. ***To instruct***: In times of emergency the public is hungry for instruction. How to act? What should or should not be done? Where can we get vaccination/gas masks/Lugol pills, etc.

M.S. Green et al. (eds.), Risk Assessment and Risk Communication Strategies in Bioterrorism Preparedness, 131–133.
© 2007 *Springer.*

2. *To educate and inform*: The public have an endless appetite for information about the topic of the day. If it is a disease, – Where can we get vaccinated? Who should be vaccinated and who should not? So on and so forth.

3. *To get the message across*: Professionals from a variety of fields, briefed by the system, can be offered as expert commentators to the various media.

4. *Talking down anxiety*: Professionals can be put up to reduce the new situation to its proper proportions. The media must be given access to information. Information should be released in real time and must be credible, up to date and appropriate to the communications medium using it (print or electronic).

1.   Useful Tools

- Press conferences/briefings
- Communiqués
- Arranging a media station at the site of the incident
- Appropriate communications devices (e.g., aerials, microwave technology)
- Regular updates
- Appointing a communications liaison officer

2.   Dangers to be Aware of:

- Giving out embarrassing and noncredible information.
- Giving out boring and unattractive information.
- Background noises.
- A harassed, crowded working environment.
- Not paying attention to scheduled broadcasting times.
- Showing inappropriate favoritism to certain media.
- Not keeping up the flow of information – if the supply fails the media will start looking for other, more available sources and there will always be other sources anxious to put out information competing with ours.
- As soon as a preliminary state of readiness has been announced, set up a "war room," preferably in the Ministry of Health's Emergency Services Division.
- A team of "commentator-pundits" should be put on notice and their "front line" put on stand-by for the first interviews to the media.
- Subcommittees should begin passing all the relevant information they have to the communications war-room.
- The director of communications for the incident should discuss with his commentary team whether to begin sending out preliminary mes-

sages to the public, and if so whether to do this by direct or indirect methods, and at what level.

- Spokesmen for the relevant hospitals may be set in readiness.
- Once permission has been given, the spokesman can put out their first communiqué.
- Weigh the possibility of holding a press conference for Israeli and foreign correspondents.
- According to how the incident unfolds, the main spokesman will issue restricted statements.
- Hospital spokesmen should arrange broadcast points for reporters.
- Each hospital should have an authorized representative, regularly updated by the war-room, who keeps the information flowing to reporters waiting at the broadcast point.

At regular intervals and as the situation requires, the communications war-room should issue instructions/guidance to its team of commentator-pundits. All of the above is to be carried out in all necessary languages.

In light of all that has been said to this point, it is clear that one of the critical elements of preparedness for emergency situations is communications and that we need to invest in this all necessary resources, particularly for our handling of the communications media. Several preparedness measures need to be taken:

1. Great amounts of information on the topic (the disease, epidemic, whatever it is) must be kept ready. A good idea is to set up a central Internet site containing as much information on the topic as can be got hold of.
2. A pool of lecturers on all subjects should be gathered, ready to be offered to the media when the time comes.
3. A 24-hour-a-day communications room should be set up, where local and foreign reporters (and hundreds of foreign correspondents can be expected to drop in on Israel when a sensational incident occurs) can be briefed, and from where they can send their material home.
4. The system should make efforts to obtain an exclusive television channel for its communications.

In this third century of the Common Era, the vital importance of the communications media is common ground between everybody, and all the more so in times of emergency. No state action – operational, diplomatic, political, or economic – can be carried out without close media coverage, without reporters asking their questions and voicing their criticism.

All this can and must be catered for, and if it is done with professional expertise, then the needs of both state security and the communications media can be satisfied.

PREVENTION STRATEGIES AND PROMOTING PSYCHOLOGICAL RESILIENCE TO BIOTERRORISM THROUGH COMMUNICATION

Anne Speckhard[*]
Adjunct Associate Professor of Psychiatry
Georgetown University Medical Center
Professor of Psychology
Vesalius College, Free University of Brussels

1. Abstract

This paper examines the challenges that governments and civil society faces in preparing for bioterrorist attacks – the challenges of reporting bioterrorism in the media, the psychological responses that are likely and how to deal with them, how terrorism may disrupt the political processes and how to respond to the needs of the population for calming, and accurate information while minimizing fear states and maximizing compliance with government instructions. It examines the psychological dimensions of mass bioterrorist attacks on the civil population and government responses, working first from the normal government expectation of panic to a more modulated recognition that even when panic does occur, such as increased attachment, cohesive, and supportive societal behaviors in response to disaster situations. Likewise, this paper addresses medical, psychiatric, psychosocial, and informational needs that are likely to be encountered in the face of "invisible" threats and makes suggestions for designing risk communication strategies to address psychological contagion, acute and posttraumatic responses, and to maximize resilience in the face of the increased bioterror threats of today's world. Today's terrorists are skillful in their manipulation of mass media to amplify the effects of their attacks. In response, governments must be equally prepared and ready to remain calm and truthful in their communication in times of crisis, and must not compromise the core values of democracy in taking up the defense against terrorism.

---

[*] Special thanks to graduate student Beatrice Jacuch who assisted in some of the background research for this paper.

M.S. Green et al. (eds.), Risk Assessment and Risk Communication Strategies in Bioterrorism Preparedness, 135–162.
© 2007 *Springer*.

2.   Introduction

Of all the weapons in the terrorist arsenal those that involve weapons of mass destruction (WMD) and those that make use of biological, radiological, or chemical threats are the most terrifying of all. Instinctively all people fear poisons and a lethal, or poisoning agent that is unseen and difficult to comprehend can quickly and easily become in the public consciousness an all pervasive threat that seems impossible to protect against even if it has touched only a small portion of the population, or is only a threatened action. Bioterrorism is terrifying not only in the mind of the ordinary citizen, but perhaps even more so in the mind of the scientist, because of the threat of death or serious and perhaps deforming illness by contagion, which spreads spontaneously beyond the original attack – through vectors the terrorists themselves cannot control. In the case of bioterrorism the agent released into society is alive and often lethal – much like the terrorists themselves – and continues to carry out their death threat beyond the original strike. In this case both the media and the biological agent itself amplify the original attack multiplying its terror causing effects. Likewise the psychological contagion that often occurs with the threat of or actuality of a bioterrorist attack is of paramount importance to consider when one looks ahead to how to promote resilience to this type of terrorism. This paper addresses the need for societies to think ahead and anticipate civilian responses to bioterrorism, to design prevention strategies, and promote resilience through communication – in the media and through governmental and nongovernmental channels. In this way society can be prepared to defend against terrorism when and if it does strike.

3.   Terrorism as a Psychological Weapon

Terrorism is essentially a psychological weapon waged upon society by unseen and sometimes even undeclared actors who attack civilian populations using various unconventional means in order to create the most horror, fear, and panic possible. In this type of psychological warfare civilians are targeted for political purposes in order to continually create and reinforce in civilian perceptions an ongoing sense of threat and dread – that anyone and anyplace, at anytime can be a victim. By achieving this aim the terrorist can force concessions, withdrawals and win on their deadly battleground. In nearly every case the terrorists' main goal is to hit the largest possible target (symbolically or in the number of casualties) and by doing so use the media to amplify its horror driven message – make your government give in to our concessions or suffer more threats to civilian security. Terrorism is used to create states of fear, horror, and dread not only in its immediate victims but in its wider witnessing audience.

The emerging threat of global terrorism is one that is dynamic and continually redefining itself in response to counterterrorism measures. The progress and portability of high-tech weaponry and the ability to communicate information quickly (over Internet and telephone) has advanced the ability of small groups to create virtual command centers that can operate simultaneously and cover multiple world regions, and in doing so enact events of worldwide mass terrorism. Moreover biological, chemical, and nuclear WMD – all previously weapons of states – are increasingly coming within the grasp of smaller groups of actors, and terrorists have made clear their desire to obtain and use such weapons.

4.   Four Tiers in the Defense Against Terrorism

In the fight against terrorism societies must prepare themselves for all variants of terrorist attack and institute policies that prevent widespread dread and panic, and promote resilience in the larger civil society.[1] The defense against terrorism is in reality four-tiered. Firstly, it involves investing huge amounts of resources into hardening defenses in terms of securing buildings, airports, and civil military installations. This defense is important in securing key resources. Yet it has been called a placebo response by some because in reality, the entire nation can be a target, total defense is illusory and any death will achieve media coverage – thereby radicalizing public opinion and demonstrating the ineffectiveness of the security forces (Mackenzie, 2006). Secondly, tier of defense against terrorism includes infiltrating and destroying terrorist groups – by discovering and thwarting their plans ahead of time and raising questions about their methods and ideology within the groups (Atran, 2003; Post, 2006).

---

[1] Civil society being broadly defined here as the formal and informal structures of society that help shape interactions amongst the population including nongovernmental organizations (NGOs), media, and those intermediary institutions (e.g., professional associations, religious groups, labor unions, citizen advocacy organizations, etc.), which build links between the population, provide information, analyses and political responses, and that give voice to various sectors of society and enrich public participation in democracies.

Of course civil society never acts in a vacuum or completely independent of government hence this paper focuses often upon how the two overlap, including through laws, policies, and instructions from one governing the other, as well as their interaction through the media, the public health service, hospitals, medical institutions, universities, think tanks, foundations, the legal system etc.

Thirdly, for winning the "war on terrorism" societies can defend against terrorism by working to understand and diminish the reasons for popular support of terrorist groups – "debranding" the ideology[2] and looking for and addressing the root causes. Lastly and most importantly for this paper is the need for society to anticipate the responses of its own citizenry to terror attacks of all kinds and build resilience into it so that the psychological effects of terrorism are minimized.

5.   The New Terrorism

5.1.   AVOWED INTEREST OF TERRORISTS IN BIOTERRORISM AND WEAPONS OF MASS DESTRUCTION

With the advent of groups like al-Qaeda and the interest in creating terror attacks involving mass casualties and the use of self martyrdom missions many in the terrorism field have begun to speak of a "new terrorism".[3] Whether or not we are seeing a real break with old terrorists' methods and goals it is certainly true that today's terrorists function in a completely new global environment. With the erosion of strict borders between countries (particularly in the European Union) and even world regions (since the fall of the Soviet bloc), the advance and portability of high-tech weaponry including biological, chemical, and nuclear hazards, and the ease and speed of communication through the Internet and telephones for purposes of recruitment, training, and planning terror attacks – terrorists now have a global playing field in which even small groups of individuals can motivate, plan, and enact mass terrorist events. Moreover biological, chemical, and nuclear WMD – all previously weapons of states – not small groups, are increasingly coming within the grasp of smaller groups of actors, and terrorists have made clear their desire to obtain and use such weapons.

The most well-known and perhaps most feared global terrorists are al-Qaeda and its affiliates. Chillingly they have avowed their willingness to use WMD including bioterrorism (Schweitzer, 2003). In addition to the much publicized words of Osama bin Laden in which he stated it was a sin not to make use of such weapons, Shamil Basayev, leader of the Chechen terrorist groups has also avowed his willingness to attack his enemies with the same agents he believes his people have been attacked with including

---

[2] I am indebted to Thelma Gillen of the UK MOD for this brilliant idea of attempting to "debrand" an ideology, much like one might attempt to debrand a trademark.

[3] Martha Crenshaw severely criticizes this conceptualization, which she credits to Simon and Benjamin.

bioterrorism.[4] Abu Musa'ab al Suri one of the contemporary al-Qaeda ideologues also advocated the use of WMD and criticized Osama bin Laden for not previously using them (Paz, 2005).[5] Likewise Aum Shinrikyo, a non-al-Qaeda linked group, that was active in Japan aimed to develop such weapons and actually shocked the world with the first mass chemical attack when they dispersed sarin gas in the Tokyo subway, injuring hundreds. Likewise two al-Qaeda affiliate groups were thwarted in their attempts to use a ricin like substance in London and Paris, and a failed biological attack was carried out in the United States when a small anti-government group attempted to contaminate a salad bar with *Salmonella*. So clearly there is an avowed willingness by today's terror groups to resort to the use of bioterrorism.

5.2.   INITIAL ADVANCES TOWARD BIOTERRORIST ATTACKS

As far as intelligence analysts have been able to piece together when groups are searching for WMD they have thus far resorted to utilizing state sponsorship, trying to buy materials on the world black market, or resorted to illicit pilferage. When these activities have not worked, terror groups have adjusted their strategies by putting their resources into internal

---

[4] Reuven Paz writes, "Abu Mus'ab al-Suri – a former leading trainer and scholar of al-Qaeda, published two significant documents calling for a new organization of Global Jihad: "The Islamist Global Resistance." One was a nine-page letter published in December 2004, and the other was a huge book totaling 1,600 pages about the strategy of Global Jihad… In his open letter to the State Department, Al-Suri talks at length about the importance of using WMD against the United States as the only means to fight it from a point of equality. He even criticizes Osama bin Laden for not using WMD in the September 11 attacks: "If I were consulted in the case of that operation I would advise the use of planes in flights from outside the U.S. that would carry WMD. Hitting the U.S. with WMD was and is still very complicated. Yet, it is possible after all, with Allah's help, and more important than being possible—it is vital." Al-Suri states that "the Muslim resistance elements [must] seriously consider this difficult yet vital direction."

[5] Reuven Paz writes, "Abu Mus'ab al-Suri – a former leading trainer and scholar of al-Qaeda, published two significant documents calling for a new organization of Global Jihad: "The Islamist Global Resistance." One was a nine-page letter published in December 2004, and the other was a huge book totaling 1,600 pages about the strategy of Global Jihad… In his open letter to the State Department, Al-Suri talks at length about the importance of using WMD against the United States as the only means to fight it from a point of equality. He even criticizes Osama bin Laden for not using WMD in the September 11 attacks: "If I were consulted in the case of that operation I would advise the use of planes in flights from outside the U.S. that would carry WMD. Hitting the U.S. with WMD was and is still very complicated. Yet, it is possible after all, with Allah's help, and more important than being possible—it is vital." Al-Suri states that "the Muslim resistance elements [must] seriously consider this difficult yet vital direction."

research and development (Hoffman, 2005). The Aum Shinrikyo group recruited and hired highly trained Russian scientists and set up a highly specialized laboratory. Likewise, information discovered in Afghanistan makes clear that al-Qaeda was engaged in a serious effort to develop a usable chemical and biological weapons capability. Seized materials include films of tests carried out by al-Qaeda operatives showing that the group achieved their goals enough to having reached the stage of limited testing of agents on live subjects. In the United Kingdom and France terrorists groups have utilized crude recipes for biological agents such as ricin (Hoffman, 2005; Schweitzer, 2003). In the thwarted UK case the group planned to smear small amounts of ricin on the door handles of random vehicles and thereby hoped to create mass hysteria from a few deaths rather than enact a mass killing.[6]

5.3. UNDERMINING PUBLIC CONFIDENCE AND CREATING MASS ANXIETY WITH BIOTERRORISM

Terrorists have certainly observed that it is possible to undermine public confidence and create mass anxiety responses by simple and even limited dispersal of a biological agent. The huge public reaction to the anthrax attacks in the United States (and indeed worldwide when one considers the number of US embassies that were also affected, as well as the many hoax attacks throughout Europe which were taken seriously by emergency providers) included: shutting down buildings; strangling the mail system; workers donning masks and rubber gloves while processing mail; quarantining areas, requiring employees to take precautionary strong antibiotics, public and private stock piling of medicines, and widespread anxiety about anthrax. These responses made clear that one could both undermine public confidence and create widespread mass distress with relatively few anthrax attacks (Hoffman, 2005; Speckhard, 2002a). Likewise the fact that it took 4 months and $41.7 million to decontaminate the Hart Senate Office Building and nearly $100 million to do the same in the Boca Raton postal facility demonstrated the high costs of responding to the dispersal of minute quantities of a biological agent. Terrorists learned from these events that rendering an important facility inoperable by virtue of biocontamination can have widespread and devastating social, psychological, and economic repercussions (Hoffman, 2005).

---

[6] The so-called Chechen cell of North Africans in Paris were discovered preparing ricin for an attack on the Russian embassy in Paris and the London group had already prepared large quantities of ricin for an unspecified attack.

During the UK trial of the al-Qaeda affiliate leaders involved in the ricin scandal it became apparent that the terrorists were more interested in their ability to undermine public confidence and to potentially create mass hysteria with a bioterrorism attack than in actually enacting a mass killing event. Likewise the Algerian cell's interest in ricin appears to be based in their inability to achieve sufficient media impact using strictly conventional attacks (Hoffman, 2005). Terrorism relies upon making a strong media impact and bioterrorism has that potential.

5.4. MASS BIOTERRORIST ATTACK MAY BE SIMPLY A MATTER OF TIME

While the war in Afghanistan made significant inroads in taking out the main al-Qaeda leadership, its ideology still flourishes and in the absence of a strong centralized leadership the movement has continued unabated. Recruitment, training and perhaps most important, a motivational ideology is daily transmitted globally via the Internet bringing on board a disparate (but unified by a common ideology) group of disenfranchised, alienated, frustrated, and even traumatized individuals living in both conflict and non-conflict zones willing to sign on to support and even enact terrorism. In terms of western security, this is particularly troublesome in Europe where radicalization among disenfranchised Muslim communities appears to be a swelling phenomenon. The unresolved conflicts and human rights violations in Chechnya, Palestine, Kashmir, and now in Afghanistan, Iraq, and Guantanamo Bay as well, all give fuel to the al-Qaeda ideology, which argues that Islam is under attack by corrupt western powers and militant jihad including attacks on civilians and self martyrdom operations is not only justified, but a duty. With the current ease of communication, lessening of technological barriers, convincing ideology, and a ready pool of recruits, it appears that the occurrence of a mass bioterrorism attack may simply be only a matter of time.

Given this state of affairs can we anticipate the responses of our citizenry to bioterrorism and if so how can government and civil society prepare and increase societal resilience to such attacks?

6.   Unrecognized Resilience in Society

To answer this question we must acknowledge that our citizenry is far more resilient than they are often given credit for. The common view espoused by government officials and policymakers is an expectation that people will panic in the face of a mass terrorist event and that chaos will ensue. Experience with terrorism, however, does not bear that out (Wessely, 2004), although most of our research is based on conventional versus bioterrorism. In nearly all civil disasters that have been studied by researchers, holding aside the moments of escaping an imminent danger such as a fire, earthquake, hurricane, or bomb – researchers repeatedly have found that citizenry has become quite attachment and community-oriented in times of threat. Total strangers help each other, open their homes, volunteer their resources, and risk their lives to help each other. Society actually becomes more civil during times of disaster as social cohesion increases rather than decreases under threat: in the short-term attachment behaviors generally increase, social cohesion increases, and the heroic is often called forth in ordinary people (Speckhard, 2005a). We have numerous studies that bear this out.

9/11 is a good example. After-the-event interviews of persons involved revealed that people did not take a "me first attitude", disabled and injured persons were not run over by panicking hordes or left behind, abandoned (Furedi, 2004). On the contrary the 9/11 evacuation was self-generated, orderly, and without panic, and those who were hurt or disabled were carefully and calmly assisted and taken to emergency services (Glass and Schoch-Spana, 2002). The explosion of the Chernobyl nuclear power plant gives us another window in which to view the responses of citizenry in times of mass disaster. When the reactor was about to explode the plant operators did not abandon their posts and flee like cowards to protect themselves. Instead they heroically fought to the last moments to shut down the reactor, to contain the damage – many giving their lives to do so. The Madrid train bombings give us another example. Witnesses state that after the first explosions passengers helped one another and calmly began to exit the scene. Only when repeated blasts occurred did some begin to run. Even then, when it became clear that emergency vehicles were having a hard time getting to the platform, taxi drivers waiting for customers did not flee in fear, but volunteered themselves as makeshift ambulances and ferried wounded persons to emergency care (Speckhard, 2004b). The same happened in the Moscow subway bombings – people walked calmly for long distances in the darkness, helping the wounded to evacuate. When terrorists bombed a crowded rock concert outside of Moscow – the band agreed to bravely play on, the audience followed instructions not to stampede in fear and the wounded were carefully attended to. In the Moscow theater where 800 hostages were held by Chechen suicide terrorists the hostages also remained calm for the most part during their ordeal and helped one another (Speckhard, 2004a; Speckhard et al., 2004; Speckhard et al., 2005a, b). Even in the Beslan hostage taking crisis where hundreds of children were held hostage, water and toilet privileges were withheld, and shooting occurred in front of the hostages – there were only limited outbreaks of hysteria. For the most part the adults present calmed the children and some extremely heroic behaviors were displayed (Speckhard, 2005c). The London public transportation bombings also met with relative calm, with Londoners quickly resuming confidence in the use of public transportation (Wessely, 2005).

Even under sustained and intense terrorist threat such as what has occurred in Israel during the second intifada (uprising) we witness that the vast majority of the population there has habituated to the threat, certainly making adjustments in daily living to avoid as much as possible their potential for being killed by terrorists – but yet carrying on with life all the same. While the psychological costs of living under a sustained and intense terror threat are still not well understood (likely causing hyperarousal states in many, bodily distress, etc.) we do also see that most of the Israeli population have on their own found ways to be resilient in the face of it. Terrorists aim at creating widespread horror, dread, and fear, and to divide society. However, it is safe to say that despite this when under threat one can see in civil society, at least in the short term that attachment behaviors generally increase, social cohesion increases, and the heroic is often called forth in ordinary people.

While this is true of terrorism that involves bombs and destruction we know less about societal responses to bioterrorism and we may find that the lessons learned from one type of terrorism may not transfer as well to another. We still have not studied well the potential effects of a mass bioterrorism event in which the dread caused by the spread of an invisible, contagious, and potentially lethal pathogen may be horrendous and in fact lead to less resilient responses. In this case the spread of horror from the terrorist attack will be amplified not only by the mass media but also by the many vectors of contagious contact all of which are difficult for ordinary individuals, much less medical professionals to understand and cope with. Likewise trying to contain a potentially lethal contagious disease, that has a presymptomatic incubating period, and that can be spread through contact with others is extremely challenging and requires societal cohesion and compliance with rapidly responding and well-informed government authorities. In this case quarantines and the means of enforcing them, panic-driven hoarding of medicines and overwhelming the medical care services with "worried well" and psychosomatic individuals are issues that we know from other disasters might well occur and, which might severely impact societal resilience. Thus we cannot say in all cases we expect society to be resilient. When it comes to poisons, invisible toxins, and fear inducing contagious illness, we have to look at other incidents to draw lessons.

7.   Fear of the Unseen and Unknown – Poisons, Toxins, Biochemical and Radiological Agents

When a threat is invisible and difficult to comprehend, some individuals may be expected to respond with fear, aggression, hysteria, and even psychosomatic symptoms if the fear of a potential toxic exposure becomes overwhelming. Such responses have been witnessed in many events and are well documented in the literature. After the Goiania radioactive incident (Brandao Mello et al., 1991), following Chernobyl (Bromet et al., 1998; Green et al., 1994; Havenaar et al., 2002; Speckhard, 2002b), and after the sarin attacks in the Tokyo subway, medical systems were briefly overwhelmed by thousands of individuals who feared that they had the symptoms of poisoning, many who became psychosomatically ill. The explosion of the Chernobyl nuclear power plant was perhaps the most serious "invisible" threat to date. Likewise the Bhopal and Goiania and other similar incidents give us additional information making clear that there are unique psychological and fear responses to "invisible" toxins, poisons, and contaminants, as well as the widespread dread of pervasive and random threat that accompanies conventional terrorism.

8.   Psychosocial Contagion

Not only is disease contagious but psychosocial phenomena can also spread as infectiously through populations as biological agents, sometimes wreaking as much havoc with health as the disease agents themselves. The processes whereby emotions, attitudes, beliefs, and behavior are spread, transmitted, and even leap between populations, similar to other contagious outbreaks like measles, chicken pox, or even the common cold is referred to as psychological or psychosocial contagion. Psychosocial contagion moves from person to person, often times requiring only a single exposure.

Categories of contagion important for understanding potential societal responses to bioterrorism include emotional, behavioral and aggression contagions. Mood, fear, and anxiety states can be transmitted quickly through a population as humans tend to synchronize their facial expressions, voices, and postures with those in their immediate environment taking on fear and distress states when they witness these in those around them (Behnke et al., 1994; Hatfield et al., 1993; Hsee et al., 1992; McDougall, 1920). This is particularly true of children. This synchronization can occur in response to viewing live footage in the mass media and may be one of the modern day mechanisms for rapid transmission of emotional contagions.

Behavioral contagions can also occur. For instance individuals exposed to violations of rules often increase their likelihood to engage in a similar or identical behaviors (i.e., speeding, delinquency, criminality, teenage smoking, youth sex, substance abuse) (Connolly, 1993; Ennett et al., 1997; Jones, 1998; Jones and Jones, 1995; Rowe et al., 1992). These two contagions – emotional and behavioral likely explain the psychology behind the hysterical buy out of duct tape in the United States when word got out that the Homeland defense report had made mention of duct tape as a useful means of protecting oneself from chemical and biological attacks. Similarly it can explain in part why many Americans were massively noncompliant and failed to heed public health officials instructions not to stockpile Cipro (flaxocin) the antibiotic used to treat anthrax, instead of following a general panic among many to buy out unnecessary antibiotics and perhaps by doing so deprive those truly in need of them. If the anthrax attacks had been widespread, this may have caused significant hardship for some.

As of this writing, we see the dread and dismay caused as Avian flu makes its way westward, with many citizens overly worried and rejecting poultry products and others noncompliant due to economic concerns of losing livelihoods, with the long-term health and economic consequences still unknown. Certainly governments must plan ahead for how they would handle issues of quarantine if it were needed and work beforehand with the public to get their participation and acceptance for plans, as well as with the media, police, military, or national guard units that would be responsible for reporting on and enforcing quarantine so that as much as possible contentious issues are dealt with and anticipated beforehand. Even rehearsing how a decontamination unit would function in a mass terror setting is important for small but crucial issues like deciding does everyone who goes through the unit have to strip naked and if so can provisions be made for segregating the sexes – a difficult issue for those for whom modesty is a key value; how do decontamination units handle the need to give up contaminated items including car keys – raising the issue of how does one get home; or how to handle the surrender of contaminated mobile phones – creating stresses and tensions for family members who can no longer check on and reassure their loved ones. Small but crucial issues like these if anticipated and thought through beforehand, with useful remedies built into the response scenarios can be arranged for the least stressful responses. New models of readiness are necessary to counter this threat especially when it pertains to biological terrorism because biological contamination raises unique and difficult issues, differing dramatically from other types of terrorism.

As psychological contagion is a very real response to the potential of toxic exposure, medical systems should prepare ahead for massive onslaughts of the "worried well". The severe acute respiratory syndrome (SARS) virus crossing from Asia to Canada in a very short time – shutting down an entire city; the Cyrptosporidium epidemic of 1993 in the state of Wisconsin; and the current epidemic with avian flu makes clear that huge number of people can be affected when a bio-threat spreads quickly through a community and that these threats raise difficult psychological and medical issues (Glaser, 2004). Governments and media must work together preparing ahead of time on how to communicate calmly in such crises in a manner that will offer useful preventative measures, minimize the potential negative effects of psychosocial contagions (including citizenry becoming noncompliant and aggressive), prevent mass sociogenic illness from occurring, and prevent overwhelming of the medical systems by those whose emotional state has put them in need of medical care. In the case of bioterrorism as we shall see this is no easy task.

9.   Mass Sociogenic Illness

In its extreme form psychosocial contagion can spawn mass hysterical contagions or mass sociogenic illness – that is, the rapid spread of illness signs and symptoms, which has no physical basis for the symptoms and no known exposure to a pathogen (Bartholomew and Wessely, 2002; Cohen et al., 1978; Kerckhoff, 1968; Marsden, 1998). Hysterical contagions involve the spread by contact, including mass media exposure, of reported symptoms and experiences usually associated with clinical hysteria (hallucinations, nausea, vomiting, fainting, etc.) in the absence of exposure to a pathogen. Such illnesses often begin with exposure of a limited group to a biological contagion or chemical toxin with the others around these persons or learning of them responding hysterically with some form of nervous excitation, including a significant loss or alteration of function, and physical symptoms with no basis in physical etiology. These types of illness often affect members of a cohesive group although they can leap across groups when common links are made in reality or imagination. Such links are often made through the mass media in which one quite limited group of individuals is actually exposed to a biological or chemical toxin and has real symptoms but other groups fear that they too have been exposed.

Study of these types of contagions has found that exposure to the verbal reporting of symptoms rather than exposure to the symptoms themselves was enough to pass it on to others (Colligan and Murphy, 1982), which makes it clear that responsible and nonhysterical news reporting is very necessary to contain such contagions. Often there is a sensitizing issue that makes populations vulnerable to psychogenic illness. In Belgium in 1999, a mass sociogenic illness occurred in response to tainted Coca Cola that gave off harmless fumes, but caused psychogenic symptoms in schoolchildren and members of the general public. This may have occurred because the Belgian public had been sensitized by serious food scares during the previous year involving dioxin contamination in the food (Nemery et al., 2002). Research has also shown that when one groups feels under attack by an enemy it is much easier for the symptoms to spread as the "victim" group finds it easy to believe that they have been poisoned by their enemies (Bartholomew and Wessely, 2002). This occurred in Palestine (Modan et al., 1983), Kosovo (Hay and Foran, 1991), and recently in Chechnya.

Recent evidence indicates people do not even have to be present at a terrorist event to experience posttraumatic symptoms (Speckhard, 2002a, b; Speckhard and Mufel, 2003). Likewise, numerous studies have shown that television coverage had a profound impact on children after the Challenger explosion (Terr et al., 1999), the first Gulf War (Cantor et al., 1993), and the Oklahoma City bombing (Pfefferbaum et al., 2000; Pfefferbaum, 2001). The impact of the 9/11 attacks was reported as far away as Italy (Apolone et al., 2002) and India (Ray and Malhi, 2005) and was acutely experienced by expatriate Americans in Belgium (Speckhard, 2002a, b; Speckhard and Mufel, 2003). In these studies, media and, particularly television exposure, was an important predictor of stress or traumatic symptoms in the face of terrorism second to geographic distance from the attacks. We must recognize that graphic images have the potential to be traumatic in themselves in terms of their potential to create a "witnessing" experience of trauma and their constant replay can also become traumatic reminders, resulting in persistent reexperiencing and hyperarousal symptoms (Hayez, 2001). Personalizing the event and reflecting on oneself as a potential victim also proved to cause stress symptoms (Dixon et al., 1993), something that can also occur via televised images.

10.   Mass Media's Role in Mediating Emotional and Behavioral Contagions

Terrorists' goals are to spread horror in behalf of their political cause and they reach their goal of maximum psychological impact through their manipulation of the mass media. The media, which is in a sense symbiotic with all the horrors of the world, generally responds within minutes of any terror attack and coverage begins immediately. In the case of a mass terror attack, the "talking heads" follow shortly thereafter. In most cases of mass terrorism it will be through these channels that the population will learn what has happened and form their attitudes about how bad it is, what the potential effects are, what they should do, and what they should fear. It is at this moment that governments can make or fail to make crucial interventions to the resiliency of civil society – by what they communicate or fail to communicate.

Journalist Robert Frank points out that in a disaster situation people often "only recall from the peak moment, in the peak intensity, and far less attention is paid to the more accurate picture that emerges over time." This then according to Frank, "creates a predisposition to think a certain way before the facts are fully presented and afterward then only to listen and retain those that confirm what was previously believed." Unfortunately journalists are under pressure to get stories quickly and report the news with insufficient information. Frank goes on to state, "It is however, very, very seductive to news-workers to appear knowledgeable when you are not" (Speckhard, 2002b).

Certainly the emotional and behavioral response of citizenry to an event of bioterrorism will depend in part on how well and calmly government communicates the events to citizens and directs them in useful activities rather than leaving an information vacuum for the media experts or "talking heads" to fill with emotionally fearful information. If governments wish to avoid such consequences and compete with the unbridled freedom of mass media to form public opinions they must be prepared and have their own "sound bites" and "talking heads" prepared well ahead of a disaster, otherwise the mass media will fill the vacuum. While the practice of journalists presenting incomplete stories with only half fashioned facts is unlikely to disappear, government and the public health systems have a responsibility to prepare ahead of time and be ready to provide psychological triage – both through the media and in person for the worried well and psychosomatic individuals who will likely overwhelm the medical facilities. In the short term government and experts credibility is crucial. Once that is lost it is very difficult to calm arousal states in individuals who will not believe competing information from that they already took on board.

Terrorists thrive on creating a mental environment in which citizens live in fear and dread of the next attack. Civil society can do a lot to fight this type of psychological tactic. One of the most important ways is for those in charge of information to be well prepared and to speak in a reassuring manner about what is both known and unknown, giving essential information but not creating a sense of constant danger. This is a difficult but necessary balance to strike.

In providing psychological reassurance over the media, government needs to think ahead of time to taking advantage of the new technologies as well – particularly the Internet. In today's world we must recognize that many people will instantly log onto the Internet in search of information and that rumors will abound. Public health officials should have already prepared and be ready to launch (or have already launched) reliable and useful information via the Internet and through all other channels of mass media to reassure the public and instruct them for the most protective responses. Likewise government can make use of mobile phones, computers, and hand held devices that can receive transmissions with messages specifically aimed at them by virtue of where they are presently located. In the case of a contagious outbreak it is possible to transmit information regarding advisories of where not to travel and information about which hospitals and clinics in the area are free versus overwhelmed and general health care advice for that regional area (Hopmeier, 2006). In this case credibility is crucial. Government must be very careful from the beginning to not lose the trust of the public in announcing what is known and still unknown, and to address psychosomatic responses in a meaningful way that differentiates them from the actual illness in question.

While state control of media is an anathema to those who hold dear the rights of free press and freedoms of speech, the media can take actions collectively to self censure sensationalist reporting that continues to ratchet up fears. Government spokespersons can put fears in perspective reminding people not to generalize from one event to all potential possibilities. For instance, following the February 2004 Moscow subway suicide bombing that killed less than 200 persons, Moscow's Carnegie Center Dmitri Trenin stated, "Every time I go down into the underground I wonder if I will finish my journey. Now nine million people feeling they are playing Russian roulette" (Ostrovsky, 2004). While this was a statement of his feelings, it reflects the sense of psychological contagion that can occur when nine million people fear an event that affected only a very small proportion of their total. Statistically the dreaded terror event is much more unlikely to happen to them than many other ordinary horrors that they forget to fear. The same occurred with the sniper in the Washington area in the fall of 2002, with fear of a deadly but highly unlikely threat nearly paralyzing a huge metropolitan area. Terrorists win when they can create a sense of dread of a pervasive and random threat – one that can strike anyone, anywhere at anytime. Invisible threats – as involved in bioterrorism have the most likelihood of achieving this goal.

11.   The Importance of Calm and Truthful Communication in Times of Crisis

The Chernobyl disaster is probably the most well-known example of an abysmal failure by government to communicate and protect its citizenry and the effects of this failure are still felt today. Twenty years later the population has still not recovered from fearing what their government failed to protect them from and many individuals disregard competing causes for illnesses such as alcoholism, pollution, stress, poor nutrition, etc., with nearly every birth defect, many serious illnesses – especially cancer, and even symptoms of minor distress in the region still suspected and blamed on Chernobyl (Speckhard, 2002b, b).

Most of the potential bioterrorist threats are clear – although the uncertainty lies as to where, when and how. Thus it is possible for government to think ahead to what the population needs to know to respond calmly and with insight. Indeed it may be wise to be already letting people know that smallpox vaccinations work even after exposure, that anthrax can be lethal upon direct exposure but is not spread infectiously. These bits of information can lay a foundation for calm responses, should the dreaded event occur, and create confidence that one could survive.

In the wake of an actual mass terror event it is wise if the government has prepared ahead of time on who will speak and given some thought, not only to the facts that must be relayed, but also to that *how* the message is relayed is often as important as the message itself. The emotional tone of the message can create fear or calm. The Israelis' success during the first Gulf War (1991) when the population was being bombarded by Scud missiles and directed to don gas masks (including putting them on small children), and retire to safe bio-sealed rooms in the event of a bioterror attack depended in large part on the preparation taken beforehand by government to disperse gas masks and to teach individuals how to take preventative measures to respond to bioterrorism. Likewise Israeli Army spokesman, Nahman Shai, whose task it was to announce to the citizenry instructions to don gas masks and go to shelters, performed this duty in such a reassuring manner that he is still remembered fondly. In providing this anxiety inducing information at the moment of imminent attack his voice remained so calm and soothing as did his demeanor that he was later nicknamed the "the valium of the nation."

Likewise when the decision was made in Israel to inoculate first responders (i.e., medical personnel, police officers, public health teams, and army soldiers) to a potential bioterrorism attack involving smallpox the fear surrounding doing so was addressed by the general director of the ministry of health, Boaz Lev, going on television and being the first to take the inoculation – showing by example that he had faith that it was worth the risks of doing so. This is a heroic example of how to communicate calmness in a crisis situation.

Often when a disaster or terrorist event occurs all the information is not known and the greatest psychological issue is about safety and what is next. Frightened citizens want to know what to expect and they need things explained in a way they can understand. This is difficult for government officials who often do not have all the information they need to respond immediately and do not know if the threat is ongoing. In this case it is of paramount importance to tell the truth. Short-term pacifications achieved with falsehood only create mistrust and blame later. It is far wiser to state clearly what is known and to admit what is still not known, making it clear that government is working hard to get the answers and nothing will be withheld to achieve maximum protection for the citizens. When explaining the risks of toxic and radioactive exposures it is important to speak in ways that put the dangers in perspective. Far more people currently die in road accidents than in terror attacks, radiation exposure also occurs normally at the dentist, while flying, etc. People can understand and respond better when risks are explained in terms of comprehensible and clear comparisons.

12. Preparation and Decision Making in the Face of Bioterrorism

Public health systems in the United States at least, have been losing funding in recent years. Without the foresight of politicians, to have made preparatory investments of resources and personnel, they may not be ready to handle a huge public health epidemic, especially one caused by bioterrorism. The equipment and training alone needed to competently handle a bioterrorism attack (in terms of rapid identification and containment) must be anticipated ahead of time and the need for a central command and control, and clear lines of communication often across many agencies must also be determined well in advance. These are lessons we have learned from other terrorist and disaster events. In the Japanese sarin attacks for instance the lack of emergency decontamination facilities and protective equipment resulted in a further secondary exposure of medical staff (135 ambulance staff and 110 staff in the main receiving hospital reported symptoms). The same occurred following Chernobyl.

In a training scenario involving multiple bombs and a potential chemical attack played out at the North Atlantic Treaty Organization (NATO) support facility in Brussels in 2005 numerous personnel who were unaware it was not a real event, were called to the scene – ambulances, bomb detonation, decontamination units, etc. who interacted with guards already present at the unit. It became clear in analyzing the exercise that the various actors could not communicate well, as the handheld radios of the emergency workers did not coordinate with those in the NATO support facility. It was also not clear who should take charge of the multiple units who converged upon the site and when the decontamination unit did not arrive (it went to another facility by accident) the entire "rescue" was delayed by hours. Likewise the ambulatory contaminated "victims" ran to ambulances who refused to take them – because they were contaminated – and then ran through the neighborhood. Had it been a real chemical or biological attack the contaminant or pathogen would likely have been widely spread.

A similar public safety exercise known as TOPOFF 2 – for "Top Officials 2," sponsored by the US Department of Homeland Safety and State designed to test and improve US domestic response to terrorist incidents, carried out a fictional simultaneous attack against Chicago using pneumonic plague and Seattle using a radiological bomb in May 2003. Similar to the NATO support facility exercise the real first responders were not alerted ahead of time that it was a fictional attack but once on the scene worked simulated crime scenes and treated volunteers pretending to be victims. Nineteen federal agencies, as well as state and local emergency responders from Illinois and Washington, as well as from Canada and the American Red Cross were involved. The exercise provided valuable lessons, including the realization that multiple control centers, numerous liaisons, and increasing numbers of response teams only complicated the emergency effort. Likewise officials noted that it was essential to monitor and correct false media reports that might have inflamed the public to panic (Miller, 2003). Certainly we know from such exercises that resources must be devoted not only to equipment but to careful planning of how to respond well technically and media-wise to terrorist threats, especially those involving radiological, biological, and chemical terrorism.

Most worrisome in a biological attack is the ability of government officials to detect unusual activity – as in new strange symptoms – and act early enough to contain the spread of lethal contagious disease within a geographical and population area in time to prevent mass casualties. This is extremely difficult to do as lethal contagious bioterrorist attacks will follow a trajectory beginning with exposure, to incubation, to latently symptomatic individuals to those who succumb and die. In the event of a biological terrorism attack public health officials working with government will be called upon to quickly identify if they are dealing with a bacteria, virus, or toxin and to identify it as quickly as possible and mount an efficient response. Since biological infections have an incubation period an efficient response could mean cordoning off those who have been exposed and who are potentially dangerous transmitters (vectors) of the disease. This could mean quarantining symptomless individuals in an effort to make sure that those who have been exposed and could, but are not necessarily proven to, be incubating disease do not spread it to others. It is unclear in a liberal democracy if government officials would be able to establish quarantines that keep people in, much less out, of a zone that has been identified as "exposed" to a lethal biological agent. In these cases one might envision in the United States, the National Guard or police troops called in to quarantine off a subpopulation of highly upset individuals who have families, cares, and responsibilities outside of the zone being quarantined (Pollack, 2006).

Certainly, in such a scenario, we can expect extremely strong fear and anxiety states to be transmitted quickly through the population and much rule-breaking behavior. Whether or not this would mount to the point of contagious aggression is unknown as it has never been well tested. We do know, however, that the contagion of aggressive behavior has been shown to operate in both local and dispersed collectives, particularly within transitory and unpredictable angry crowds (mobs) (Bandura, 1973; Lachman, 1996; Reicher, 1984) and we know from the recent riots in the Islamic world that such aggressive contagions can easily be mediated and whipped up by the mass media.

It is unlikely that democratic governments would ever desire or strive to shut down media reporting of a bioterrorist attack, yet we can learn from other societies that have taken this tact. After the initial stages of the Beslan hostage-taking siege, Ossetian authorities shut down broadcasts from the local televisions stations in an effort to defuse some of the local tension of televised broadcasting of the event. Likewise psychiatric consultants brought in to help with the siege realized that mothers sitting at home with nothing more to do than agitate and shame their husbands for not going to rescue their children caught in the school building had to be addressed. They organized meaningful tasks for the mothers and opened a briefing center where every three hours or so they gave reports to the townspeople outlining everything they knew about the siege, potential negotiations, the state of the children inside, and so on. While it is unlikely that western countries would follow suit in shutting down television broadcasting, and even in Beslan, cable networks, Internet, and radio continued to broadcast in the area, it is useful to think ahead on how to work with the media and how to give citizens useful tasks to help them be empowered to be heroic in a crisis versus feeling helpless and frustrated with a sense of powerless inactivity.

Government decisions on when and what to tell, regarding attempts to contain the threat using quarantine strategies, whether or not to take action in a bioterrorism attack during the period of incubation when there are still no casualties, how to educate now and during the crisis, decisions about putting resources into the public health system, making sure medicines and vaccinations are available and dispersed fairly – are all public policy issues that should be ethically addressed well ahead of time. Active public participation in such plans creates a societal investment in carrying them out. If this work has not been done ahead of time it may result in less complaint, less cohesive, and less resilient responses to terrorist threats.

13.   Psychological Triage for Acute and Posttraumatic Stress

While civilians are more resilient that given credit for, a proportion of individuals will predictably suffer from symptoms of acute and posttraumatic stress when exposed to violence and death in a terrorist attack. While many of these responses are short-lived and resolve themselves through normal coping channels, some do not. The nature of a bioterrorism event, however, is less likely to result in acute posttraumatic stress states (unless there are massive numbers of deaths) than one might expect when the attack involves an explosion or other act of mass violence because the traumatic stressor is *information* versus a witnessed trauma. This is the difficulty inherent in dealing with "invisible" stressors, such as toxins, pathogens, and contaminants – they create fear, horror, and dread but there is often no clearly defined event to address, but instead an amorphous and undefined emotional horror.

Acute stress responses to a bioterrorism attack are much more likely to include psychosocial and behavioral contagions including hysteria, somatization, mass sociogenic illness outbreaks, and hysterical and possibly even aggressive demands for medical care, vaccines, and medicines than the acute posttraumatic responses often seen in response to an explosion or an act of violence. In all cases reassuring information and calm responses are the most helpful. There is a strong body of literature that demonstrates that intrusive psychological debriefing applied in a coercive manner in the immediate aftermath of traumas, is neither necessary or helpful, and sometimes even harmful, as most acute and posttraumatic symptoms to terror attacks decline overtime when normal coping channels are utilized (National Institute of Mental Health, 2002). However, this is not to say that the "worried well" or psychosomatic individuals who appear asking for help should not receive psychological triage.

In most cases traumatized individuals and those in high arousal states will respond well to having their posttraumatic and acute stress symptoms normalized – learning that it is a normal reaction to a traumatic event to feel fear, to even be dissociative if the fear is overwhelming, to experience intrusive thoughts and bodily arousal afterwards, and to engage avoidance strategies to little avail. Learning that these are normal responses to trauma often helps individuals to move beyond them more easily versus get caught up in additional fears and shame over why they are not feeling or acting normal, as well as to diminish the avoidance responses that often occur in those who suffer from posttraumatic reexperiencing (Speckhard, 2002a; Speckhard et al., 2005a, b). Likewise those who have "caught" contagious psychological states and somatic symptoms are often also well served to receive medical care assuring them they are not a victim of the biological contaminate, as well as reassuring them that it is normal for some individuals to "catch" fear states and for these to evidence themselves in the body. In this way the individual is not shamed by having somatized their stress, something most individuals find distressing in itself, but also receives a logical explanation for what is happening in their body – an explanation that if judged as credible (and this is crucial) allows them to calm the bodily arousal that is supporting the negative symptoms. When a sense of humor and normality is introduced, the somatizing response often lessens.

However if the person's real concerns are not taken seriously, and are ridiculed, he is accused of making up symptoms, ignored or told to go home as nothing is wrong, symptoms can often worsen. Fear states can increase causing further somatization, shame can lead to strong avoidance, and isolation responses or the fear can drive aggressive responses. Thus a balance must be struck between kindly understanding gentle humor to help somatizing individuals to understand how psychological contagions pass between persons, and firm reassurance that they are indeed not infected by the biocontaminate. Of course those who are most distressed and less responsive to short-term triage should be identified and put in contact with helping professionals for longer term care with particular emphasis on those who are seriously dissociative and children with strongly embedded somatic symptoms.

The best ways to ensure that acute stress responses to a mass terrorist event are minimized is to move survivors as quickly as possible to safety and reunite family members. This can be complicated in the event of a bioterror attack as it can be unclear for sometime if it is safe for persons to be reunited and it takes some time to establish when the critical period of attack (and ensuing contagion) is over. Communications in all terror attack scenarios should be calm and clear and everything supportive that can be done to lower physiological states of arousal should be done.

We know that a natural antidote to traumatic experience is attachment – the neurobiology of the latter antagonizes the former – calming and lowering hyperarousal states. Hence behaviors that are attachment oriented – calling family, seeking out contact with others, etc. should be encouraged in the aftermath of a terror event. The Internet may also prove to be a very useful tool in this regard. Following 9/11, numerous researchers made use of the Internet as a research tool and surprisingly found it also functioned as a therapeutic tool – that discussing the issues for many functioned as a social buffer.

In terms of posttraumatic sequelae to bioterrorism there are unique long-term variants that must be taken into account. Those exposed to poisons, invisible toxins, radiation, and so forth often worry less about their "traumatic" exposure, since that was often a non-event for them at the time it occurred, but only took on importance retrospectively when they learned horrifying information about their potential exposure to a deadly contaminant or toxin, which now threatens to poison their entire future. Since horrifying information is usually the central aspect of contamination stressor and there is often an absence of sensory details in the threat, the stressor may be said to be of a more cognitive, but equally horrifying form.

Indeed, victims of toxic disasters often experience horror in their imaginations of the future. For instance, the Chernobyl victim who has a high radiation exposure as a child may continually see himself in the future as a cancer victim, or the pregnant woman exposed to a toxic contaminant may continually flash forward to the birth of deformed child, fearing to continue her pregnancy but loath to abort it. As a result survivors of toxic traumas develop a unique trauma-induced time distortion that is better understood as a "flash-forward" because it is the constant intrusion and reexperience in the mind of a horrifying, inescapable, and life-threatening event that the survivor *expects to happen in the future* as a result of having been exposed to a contaminant in the past. These flash-forwards are made up of repetitive and intrusive thoughts and images (similar to flashbacks) and create acute emotional distress and bodily agitation similar to the hyperaroused state typically observed with flashbacks (Speckhard, 2002b, 2005b). This was quite common among those traumatized by Chernobyl. They did not evidence clear posttraumatic arousal states to the memories of actual exposure but instead displayed them in response to involuntary horrific thinking about the *future*, experiencing intrusive and distressing states about getting cancer, dying young, bearing deformed children, etc. (Speckhard, 2002b, 2005b).

14.   Support for Vulnerable Populations

There are also vulnerable populations to consider in a bioterrorist attack. Pregnant women are often overlooked in such situations even though pregnancy is known to often be a time fraught with worry about the health of the future child. One researcher wrote that the highest death toll from the Chernobyl disaster was not caused by direct exposure to radiation but due to the huge increase in voluntary abortion following it, even in areas in Europe not directly exposed (Knudsen, 1991). Likewise makeshift abortions were provided for many women in the direct exposure area. The decision to abort is an extremely difficult one for many persons, particularly those with a wanted pregnancy and in instances following toxic exposure is often made in a relatively short time period with the potential for deep psychological distress afterward including impacted grief, guilt, and traumatic responses (Speckhard and Mufel, 2003; Speckhard and Rue, 1993). Given that we can anticipate many of the bioterrorist threats we may face, we should prepare ahead of time, reassuring and giving accurate information concerning the potential desire to abort what may be a perfectly healthy pregnancy, so that unnecessary abortions of wanted pregnancies do not take place.

Researchers of toxic disasters often find that mothers are often more worried about their children's symptoms than children themselves (Bromet et al., 1998). Finding a way to reach out to mothers and reassure them while giving them useful strategies for finding mastery for combating their fears, versus feeling powerless to protect their children, can also be very helpful. Likewise we must address long-term fears of mothers-to-be when contamination of any type has occurred. Girls and young women yet to bear children are often stigmatized after toxic exposures. Not only do they often fear having deformed children, even many years afterwards, but they also often become the victims of the stigmatizing fears of others, which can diminish their ability to find suitable marriage partners. Following Chernobyl, the birthrate in contaminated areas as opposed to noncontaminated areas fell dramatically from 1991 to 2001; an effect which was attributed, as most likely, due to maternal anxiety about birth defects (World Health Organization, 2005) and many young men and women who had been exposed found they were shunned as marriage partners. Worries of being exposed to a toxin, contaminant, or pathogen especially in girls and young women and in regard to childbirth nearly always is an issue that must be addressed even long after the fact of exposure.

Health-care workers are another vulnerable population. They form the front line in an often terrifying scenario caring for individuals who may contaminate them as well. They bravely risk their own health, which many are willing and able to do by virtue of their training, but this can be especially difficult for health-care workers who are also parents, or who have elderly relatives at home, and who fear exposing their own families. Indeed when the Israelis decided to inoculate their first responders against smallpox the only fatality was a family member of a doctor who ended up infecting his immune-suppressed wife. The horror of potentially contaminating one's own children was voiced by health-care workers after the SARS outbreak, as well as by those caring for contaminated individuals directly after the Chernobyl explosion, with workers saying that was the hardest part of the ordeal for them. We must take into account these very difficult situations our health-care workers will face, and consider ahead of time emergency protocols for childcare for those who take the very front lines in a serious bioterrorism threat, so that they can devote their complete energies to medical care and worry less about spreading lethal and not well understood disease at home. We must also find ways to support and honor heroic health-care workers like those who died taking care of SARS patients, as well as those others who volunteered to help with the SARS outbreak, knowing full well that to do so might be risking their lives.

In the face of a massive bioterrorism threat we should give some thought to preparing psychological triage workers – mental health workers who have been trained ahead of time to sort through psychosomatic symptoms versus those needing immediate quarantine and treatment. Given the thousands of psychosomatic and worried individuals who have overtaken the health-care systems in other similar situations, mental health-care workers can ease the burden on health-care workers and send the worried and hysterical patients home with some calming reassurance, sorting through those who also should be referred for additional psychological assistance.

15.   Not Losing What We Value Most

Terrorists achieve their goals when they manage to derail political processes and move democracies to compromise their cherished values. As many terrorist attacks have been aimed at and timed with elections it is wise for governments to plan ahead how to respond when a candidate is killed, when a terror attack occurs during an election and so forth, so that the processes of democracy do not become derailed. The chaos of a bio-terror attack can easily disrupt an election if voters are afraid to congregate in public places. It is wise to have thought ahead of time what the strategy would be for delaying or recounting an election in such a scenario.

Likewise when terrorists exploit the freedoms of liberal democracies it is tempting to surrender civil liberties in order to stop them. While some liberties may have to be suspended to effectively fight terrorism, it is important to recognize that going too far in this direction – detaining thousands of aliens following 9/11, practicing "torture lite" in detention centers, such as at Guantanamo Bay, abusing prisoners in Abu Ghraib, etc. simply discredits our integrity and plays into the terrorist promoting ideologies that support violent responses against our abuses. These things unleash the terrorists' justifications for "defending" themselves through the use of WMD including bioterrorism. We need to always occupy the higher ground and continually remind, especially those who support the new "religiously" oriented terrorists, that Islam in particular does not condone killing by poison and that many scholars of the Koran takes a firm stance against the use of such weapons. But such statements fall on deaf ears if we ourselves are guilty of similar violations of morality and ethics.

Individuals need to feel that their world is somewhat predictable and that they have some mastery in it. Bioterrorism involves an invisible threat that can create the opposite feelings: fear, horror, and dread as the actual contaminate spreads by biological contagion, and fear states including psychosomatic responses spread via psychosocial contagion. To defend against bioterrorism government initiatives should have been well thought out ahead of time, include preparatory education and a participatory process of the citizenry, preparation of experts who will be called on to help and work ahead of time with the media who will report the crisis, coupled with leaders whose words and actions inspire the belief that government is credible, calm, and acting in the public's behalf during a crisis. When leaders are honest, communicate calmly, and have prepared their societies ahead of time to respond well to terrorism, we can expect resilient responses. In times of threat and disaster populations often become attachment oriented and cohesive and heroic behaviors are frequently displayed.

The best defense against terrorism, however, is to address first and foremost the root causes of it and end the motivations of terrorist leaders and sympathizers to kill and destroy. Ultimately terrorism will not disappear until its root causes are addressed. Social injustices that inflame terrorist rhetoric must be addressed as we all work for peace and security in this new uncertain world. Until we achieve the ability to undermine terrorism by addressing its root causes, infiltrating terrorist groups and hardening our defenses we will have to continue to work toward strengthening civil society to be resilient to face this continuing threat. In the absence of achieving this we must prepare our societies with well thought out plans to be as resilient as possible.

References

1. Atran S. Genesis of suicide terrorism. Science, p. 299, 2003.
2. Bandura A. Aggression: a social learning analysis. Englewood Cliffs, NJ: Prentice-Hall, 1973.
3. Bartholomew RE, Wessely S. Protean nature of mass sociogenic illness. From possessed nuns to chemical and biological terrorism fears. Br J Psychiatry 2002; 180: 300–306.
4. Behnke PR, Sawyer CR, King PE. Contagion theory and the communication of public speaking state anxiety. Communication Education 1994; 43: 246–251.
5. Brandao Mello CE, Oliveria AR, Carvalho AB. The psychological effects of the goiania radiation accident on the hospitalized victims. In Picks RC, Berger ME, O'Hara FM Jr (ed.). The medical basis for radiation accident preparedness iii the psychological perspective. New York: Elsevier, pp. 121–129, 1991.
6. Bromet EJ, Carlson G, Goidgaber D, Gluzman S. Health effects of the chernobyl catastrophe on mothers and children. In Green B.L. (ed.). Toxic contamination: the interface of psychological and physical health effects, XIV annual meeting of the International Society for Traumatic Stress Studies, Washington, DC, 1998.
7. Cohen BGF, Colligan MJ, Wester II W, Smith MJ. An investigation of job satisfaction factors in an incident of mass psychogenic illness at the workplace. Occupational Health Nursing, January, 10–16, 1978.
8. Colligan MJ, Murphy LR. A review of mass psychogenic illness in work settings. In Colligan MJ, Pennebaker JW, Murphy LR (ed.). Mass psychogenic illness. New Jersey: Erlbaum, pp. 171–182, 1982.
9. Connolly T, Aberg L. Some contagion models of speeding. Accid Anal Prev 1993; 25: 57–66.
10. Ennett ST, Flewelling RL, Lindrooth RC, Norton EC. School and neighborhood characteristics associated with school rates of alcohol, cigarette, and marijuana use. J Health Soc Behav 1997; 38: 55–71.
11. Furedi F. Heroes of the hour. New Sci 2004; 182: 19.
12. Glaser R. We are not immune: influenza, SARS, and the collapse of the public health. Harpers Magazine July: 35–42, 2004.
13. Glass T, Schoch-Spana M. Bioterrorism and the people: how to vaccinate a city against panic. Clin Infect Dis 2002; 34: 217–223.
14. Green BL, Lindy JD, Grace MC. Psychological effects of toxic contamination. In Ursano RJ, McCaughey BG, Fullerton CS (eds). Individual and community responses to trauma and disaster: the structure of human chaos. Cambridge: Cambridge University Press, pp. 154–176, 1994.
15. Hatfield E, Cacioppo JT, Rapson RL. Emotional contagion. Cambridge: Cambridge University Press, 1993.
16. Havenaar JC, Julie G, Bromet EJ. Epilogue: lessons learned and unresolved issues in toxic turmoil: psychological and societal consequences of ecological disasters. In Havenaar J, Bromet E, Cwikel J (eds). Toxic turmoil: psychological and societal consequences of ecological disasters. New York: Kluwer Academic/ Plenum, pp. 259–273, 2002.

17. Hay A, Foran J. Yugoslavia: poisoning or epidemic hysteria in kosovo? The Lancet 1991; 338: 1196.
18. Hoffman B. Terrorism and the chemical, biological, radiological, nuclear (CBRN) threat. MIT Lecture Series, Cambridge, MA, 5 December 2005.
19. Hopmeier, M. Risk communication and psychological impact; technological and operational methods of mitigation. In Green MS, Zenilman J, Cohen D (eds). Risk assessment and risk communication strategies in bioterrorism preparedness, 2006.
20. Hsee CK, Hatfield E, Chemtob C. Assessments of the emotional states of others - conscious judgements versus emotional contagion. J Soc Clin Psychol 1992; 11: 119–128.
21. Jones MB. Behavioral contagion and official delinquency: epidemic course in adolescence. Soc Biol 1998; 45: 134–142.
22. Jones MB, Jones DR. Preferred pathways of behavioural contagion. J Psychiatr Res 1995; 29: 193–209.
23. Kerckhoff AC, Back KW. The June bug: a study in hysterical contagion. New York: Appleton-Century-Crofts, 1968.
24. Knudsen LB. Legally induced abortions in Denmark after chernobyl. Biomedicine Pharmocother 1991; 45: 229–231.
25. Lachman SJ. Psychological perspective for a theory of behavior during riots. Psychol Rep 1996; 79: 739–744.
26. Mackenzie A . Terrorism and the placebo response. Jane's Defense Weekly, February 8, 2006.
27. Marsden P. Memetics and social contagion: two sides of the same coin? Journal of Memetics: Evolutionary Models of Information Transmission 1998; 2.
28. McDougall W. The group mind. New York: Knickerbocker Press, 1920.
29. Miller C. Communicating at topoff 2: a keystone in terrorism response. Police and Security News 2003; 19(4).
30. Modan B, Tirosh M, Weissenberg E, Acker C, et al. The arjenyattah epidemic. A mass phenomenon: Spread and triggering factors. The Lancet 1983; 2: 1472–1474.
31. National Institute of Mental Health. Mental health and mass violence: evidence-based early psychological intervention for victims/survivors of mass violence: NIH publication No. 02-5138, 2002.
32. Nemery B, Fischler B, Boogaerts M, Lison D, Willems J. The coca-cola incident in Belgium, June 1999. Food Chem Toxicol 2002; 40(11): 1657–1667.
33. Ostrovsky A . Russian authorities blame Chechens as Moscow subway train blast kills 39. Financial Times, p. 6, February 7, 2004.
34. Paz R. Global jihad and WMD: between martyrdom and mass destruction. In Fradkin H, Haqqani H, Brown E (eds). Current trends in Islamist ideology, Vol. 2, Washington DC: Hudson Institute: Center on Islam, Democracy, and The Future of the Muslim World, pp. 74–86, 2005.
35. Pollack M. Risk communication and the community response to a bioterrorist attack. In Green MS, Zenilman J, Cohen D (eds). Risk assessment and risk communication strategies in bioterrorism preparedness, 2006.

36. Post J. Social and psychological factors in the genesis of terrorism. In Victoroff J (ed.).Amsterdam: IOS Press, 2006.
37. Reicher SD. The St. Paul's riot: an explanation of the limits of crowd action in terms of a social identity model. Eur J Soc Psychol 1984; 14: 1–21.
38. Rowe DC, Chassin L, Presson CC, Edwards D, Sherman SJ. An epidemic model of adolescent cigarette-smoking. J Appl Soc Psychol 1992; 22: 261–285.
39. Schweitzer Y. The age of non-conventional terrorism. Strategic assessment 6, No 1, May 2003.
40. Speckhard A. Innoculating resilience to terrorism: acute and posttraumatic stress responses in US military, foreign & civilian services serving overseas after September 11 2002a; 8(2): 105–122.
41. Speckhard A. Voices from the inside: psychological responses to toxic disasters. In Havenaar J, Bromet E, Cwikel J (eds). Toxic turmoil: psychological and societal consequences of ecological disasters. New York: Kluwer Academic/ Plenum, pp. 217–236, 2002b.
42. Speckhard A. Soldiers for god: a study of the suicide terrorists in the Moscow hostage taking siege. In McTernan O (ed.) The roots of terrorism: contemporary trends and traditional analysis. Brussels: NATO Science Series, 2004a.
43. Speckhard A. Unpublished interviews from the Madrid training bombings, 2004b.
44. Speckhard A. Civil society's response to mass terrorism: building resilience. In Gunaratna R (ed.). Combating terrorism: military and non military strategies. Singapore: Eastern Universities Press, 2005a.
45. Speckhard A. Psycho-social and physical outcomes of technological disaster: information as a traumatic stressor. In Berkowitz N (ed.). A chernobyl reader. Madison: University of Wisconsin Press, 2005b.
46. Speckhard A. Unpublished Beslan interviews, 2005c.
47. Speckhard A, Mufel N. Universal responses to abortion? Attachment, trauma and grief responses in women following abortion. J Prenat Perinat Psychol Health 2003; 18(1): 3–38.
48. Speckhard A, Rue V. Complicated mourning: dynamics of impacted post abortion grief. J Prenat Perinat Psychol Health 1993; 8; 5–32.
49. Speckhard A, Tarabrina N, Krasnov V, Akhmedova K. Research note: observations of suicidal terrorists in action. Terrorism and Political Violence 2004; 16(2): 305–327.
50. Speckhard A, Tarabrina N, Krasnov V, Mufel N. Posttraumatic and acute stress responses in hostages held by suicidal terrorists in the takeover of a Moscow theater. Traumatology 2005a; 11(1).
51. Speckhard A, Tarabrina N, Krasnov V, Mufel N. Stockholm effects and psychological responses to captivity in hostages held by suicidal terrorists. Traumatology 2005b; 11(2).
52. Wessely S. Report on the NATO Russia advisory panel on mitigating the social and psychological consequences of chemical, biological and radiological terrorism. Paper presented at the NATO headquarters council meeting, 2004.
53. Wessely S. Victimhood and resilience. N Engl J Med 2005; 353(6): 548–550.
54. World Health Organization. Health effect of the chernobyl accident and special health care programmes, 2005.

RISK COMMUNICATION AND THE COMMUNITY RESPONSE TO A BIOTERRORIST ATTACK: THE ROLE OF AN INTERNET-BASED EARLY WARNING SYSTEM A.K.A. "THE INFORMAL SECTOR"

Marjorie Pollack
ProMED-mail, International Society for Infectious Diseases, Boston, MA, USA

1. Introduction

Most agencies involved in disease surveillance and response to outbreaks, both natural and unnatural, agree that no single system provides the necessary information that will lead to timely reports of unusual health events. Current discussions point toward the need for a "network of networks" to provide wide coverage into the community for early alerts of these unusual health events. ProMED-mail is an example of an entity operating in the "informal sector" and demonstrates how it can assist in the early communication of new or ongoing disease risks not only to the health-care community, but also the interested community at large, through a moderated Internet-based listserv with a worldwide coverage [1, 2].

The formal health sector has traditionally relied upon reports of disease received through established surveillance systems in which the information travels up the familiar health pyramid (see Figure 1).

According to the above model, the events leading up to an official report on disease occurrence requires multiple steps until the first notification to the formal sector occurs. A local health facility sends a report (usually on a weekly basis) to the next level of attention (county or district level). This level then sends a weekly report to the state or provincial level, which in turn sends a report to the national level. Finally, the national level will send a report to the international level, usually the regional office of the World Health Organization (WHO), which forwards it to WHO headquarters in Geneva.

One of the challenges to getting these reports moving quickly is difficulty in communication between the health facility and the corresponding next higher level for reporting. Another key challenge arises when the person(s) who is ill does not go to an official or governmental health sector facility for the first line of care. In many areas there are private

M.S. Green et al. (eds.), Risk Assessment and Risk Communication Strategies in Bioterrorism Preparedness, 163–175.
© 2007 *Springer.*

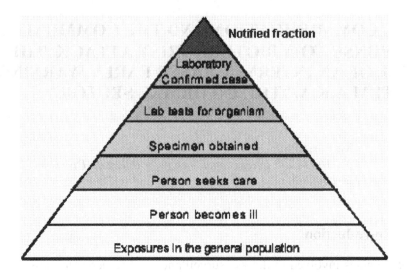

Figure 1. Communicable disease surveillance pyramid [3].

health-care providers, some formally trained, others informally trained, who provide care but are not part of the official reporting network. Hence, the official sector often does not learn about these cases until long after when they first present for treatment.

Recognizing the limitations confronting the formal health sector, especially in the domain of communication of possible disease problems, the Program to Monitor Emerging Diseases, better known as ProMED was formed in 1994. ProMED-mail is a global electronic reporting system, open to all sources, for outbreaks of emerging infectious diseases and diseases resulting from toxin exposure. It is a moderated listserv that covers plant, animal, and human diseases. Subscriptions are free, and there is a freely accessible website at: http://www.promedmail.org. ProMED-mail is a program activity of the International Society of Infectious Diseases and is a not-for-profit, non-governmental organization (NGO). This independent status permits ProMED to function without political constraints. (This translates into the ability to post reports without requiring the permission of a government to do so.)

At the time of this workshop (June 2005), there were more than 33,000 subscribers to ProMED-mail from more than 150 countries. ProMED-mail postings are reproduced on numerous other listservs and it is estimated that postings will reach approximately 100,000 computers each day. All reports posted on ProMED-mail are screened by expert moderators. Fields of expertise of the moderators include viral, bacterial, fungal, and parasitic diseases; epidemiology and surveillance; entomology; and veterinary and plant diseases.

Posted reports come from a variety of sources. Official, "formal sector" reports from regional, national, and international public health authorities are often posted to provide official confirmation of an outbreak or unusual health event.

However, the use of the "informal sector" is crucial for the acquisition of information or reports on unusual health events as they are occurring. The two main sources are lay press reports and anecdotal reports submitted by subscribers. The subscriber base in over 150 countries constitutes an international network of individuals with access to information on unusual health events (see Figure 2 for a map of ProMED-mail subscribers).

ProMED-mail subscribers include members of the international official (governmental) sector: the WHO and its regional offices, the Food and Agricultural Organization of the United Nations (FAO), and the World Animal Health Organization (OIE). There are Ministry of Health and Ministry of Agriculture personnel at the national level. It also includes members of the scientific community (at the project or field level, at the organizational level, including NGOs, and at the academic level) and non-scientific community, including members of the lay press. Often, although the official health sector may not as yet have seen cases of new diseases of concern, the lay press publishes reports on these outbreaks. ProMED-mail staff and subscribers search the Internet for such reports and post them on the listserv.

With subscribers in more than 150 countries, reports of unusual health events in one country serve as an alert for "astute clinicians" in other countries. The public health arena recognizes the important role of the astute clinician in identifying new geographic spread of diseases.

ProMED-mail focuses on the coverage of newly described or undiagnosed diseases, outbreaks, epidemics of known infectious diseases, and the emergence of known diseases in newly defined geographic areas or among newly defined populations. This applies to human diseases as well as animal and plant diseases. Animal diseases covered include zoonotic diseases with known or suspected human disease potential, as well as purely animal diseases for their ultimate impact on economies and that pertaining to food security. Similarly, plant diseases are covered for their known impact on human health as well as for economic and food security issues (Table 1). Estimates are that more than 70% of newly emerging diseases are zoonotic in origin, resulting in "species jump" from animal to humans [1, 4]. Recent examples of this include the severe acute respiratory syndrome (SARS), avian influenza, Nipah virus encephalitis, spongiform encephalopathies, and monkeypox.

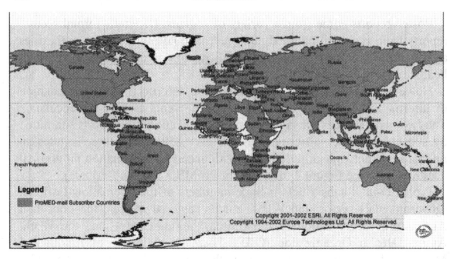

Figure 2. Map of countries with ProMED-mail subscribers.

TABLE 1. Number of ProMED-mail reports, 1994–2005, by disease, for the 18 most the ommonly reported diseases*

Disease	No. of reports
West Nile virus	831
Dengue	818
Avian influenza	746
Foot and mouth disease	744
Bovine spongiform encephalopathy	695
Cholera	684
Rabies	668
Anthrax	599
Unknown illness	563
Ebola	474
Escherichia coli O157	454
New variant Creutzfeldt–Jakob-disease	405
Salmonella	376
Hantavirus	336
Yellow fever	326
Influenza	323
Malaria	322
SARS	249

* As of 5 June 2005.

2.   Examples of use of Informal Sector

Examples of increased response by the health community to heightened disease surveillance needs facilitated through the informal sector can be seen in the reporting of four recent outbreaks.

2.1.   SEVERE ACUTE RESPIRATORY SYNDROME (SARS)

On 10 February 2003, the following posting appeared on ProMED-mail:

> PNEUMONIA – CHINA (GUANGDONG): REQUEST FOR INFORMATION
>
> **
>
> Date: 10 Feb 2003
> From: Stephen O. Cunnion, MD, PhD, MPH
>
> This morning I received this e-mail and then searched your archives and found nothing that pertained to it. Does anyone know anything about this problem?
>
> "Have you heard of an epidemic in Guangzhou? An acquaintance of mine from a teacher's chat room lives there and reports that the hospitals there have been closed and people are dying"[5].

This report was the first public notification of an outbreak in southern China of a disease that was later called SARS. By the end of the outbreak in July 2003, 8,096 probable cases of SARS had been reported with 774 deaths [6].

For the first month, after the outbreak, there were numerous reports and rumors from China about an epidemic of a severe, "atypical" pneumonia. On 11 March 2003, there was a ProMED-mail posting reporting an illness with similar symptoms in a businessman visiting Hanoi, followed by similar illnesses among hospital staff that had cared for him [7]. On 14 March 2003, ProMED-mail had received the following email from an infectious disease physician in Ontario, Canada (unpublished e-mail):

> We have an unidentified severe respiratory illness cluster in a family, one of whom was in Hong Kong 14 days ago. Can you update me on what the illness cluster in Hanoi is please?

The family cluster described in the above e-mail were the index cases for the outbreak of SARS in Ontario, Canada that by its end had affected 251 individuals with 43 deaths. This e-mail is an excellent example of an astute clinician seeing cases of a new disease that appeared similar to reports of cases occurring on the other side of the world.

The physicians in Ontario published their experiences with SARS and credited Internet-based reporting for its impact on disease identification and containment:

The identification of SARS in Canada only a few weeks after an outbreak on another continent exemplifies the ease with which infectious agents can be transmitted in this era of international travel. It also demonstrates the importance and value of information and alert systems such as the Department of Communicable Disease Surveillance Response of the World Health Organization [WHO] and the Disease Outbreak News Web site (http:// www.who.int/csr/don) and the ProMED-mail (Program for Monitoring Emerging Diseases) reporting network sponsored by the International Society for Infectious Disease (http:// www.promedmail.org) [1; 8, page 2003].

The sequence of events leading up to the worldwide alert about SARS clearly demonstrates the value of the informal sector in early disease alerts:

10 Feb 2003 – Reports of atypical pneumonia in Guangdong China – Source: ProMED subscriber, plus newswire report (Chinese) – (*informal sector*).

11 Feb 2003 – Confirmation of atypical pneumonia in Guangdong China – Source: Official WHO report (*formal sector*), newswires (*informal sector*).

11 Mar 2003 – Reports of undiagnosed respiratory illness in hospital in Hanoi VietNam – Source: Newswire (*informal sector*).

14 Mar 2003 – Reports of atypical pneumonia in East Asia – Hong Kong, Vietnam, Singapore, China (Guangdong Province), Taiwan, and Ontario Canada – Source: Official (WHO, HK DOH, CDC Taiwan) (*formal sector*) hospital staff, newswires (*informal sector*).

15 Mar 2003 – Reports of SARS worldwide – Source: WHO advisory/alert (*formal sector*).

2.2.   AVIAN INFLUENZA

The public health community clearly acknowledges that we are long overdue for a human influenza pandemic. It has long been theorized that new human influenza strains evolve as species jumps by avian influenza viruses, which through genetic reassortment obtain human-to-human transmissibility genes [9]. The appearance of a new strain of avian influenza associated with human illness has been a serious concern on the part of the public health community, as a possible precursor to the next human influenza pandemic. The following report was posted on ProMED-mail on 20 August 1997:

> **INFLUENZA, BIRD-TO-MAN, FIRST CASE?**
> **
>
> Date: Wed, 20 Aug 1997
> From: Emil Mikhles
> Subject: Influenza Strain – Hong Kong
>
> The press reported today, Aug.20 1997, that a 3-year-old boy died after contracting an influenza strain that has never been seen in humans. A specimen from the boy's trachea was identified as "influenza A of H4N1* strain," which is known to be found mainly in birds" [10]
>
> * This was corrected to be H5N1 the following day [11].

This report focused worldwide attention on the possibility that H5N1 would be the next pandemic influenza strain. At that time, H5N1 had been identified in poultry in live markets in Hong Kong and it was speculated that there were ongoing unreported outbreaks of H5N1 on the Chinese mainland [12]. During the early stages of the SARS outbreak, there were two cases of confirmed human illness with H5N1 among family members who had traveled from Fujian Province in China to Hong Kong, where their illness was diagnosed; a third suspected case was a family member who died while still in Fujian Province [13].

Following these human cases, the public health community followed the H5N1 activity in both avian and human populations. The avian H5N1 had first been identified in a goose in China in 1996 [14]. The next official report of an outbreak of H5N1 in avians was in Hong Kong, following the identification of a human case of H5N1 [15].

Following these events, there were no official reports of H5N1 activity until 2004. Early reports of suspected avian influenza outbreaks were appearing in the informal sector, as seen below:

> **AVIAN INFLUENZA – INDONESIA: REQUEST FOR INFORMATION**
> **
>
> Date: 18 November 2003
> From: ProMED-mail <promed@promedmail.org>
>
> ProMED-mail has received a report from a reliable source of rumors of the occurrence of an outbreak of avian influenza in domestic fowl in Indonesia (West Java and Sumatra). The accounts of the rumored outbreak emanate from 2 independent sources.
>
> Further information from any informed person or organization in the area would be appreciated [Mod.CP] [16]

The reliable source providing this report was a veterinarian working in the affected area, who was concerned about political and professional reper-cussions for publicly reporting this outbreak. Job security concerns are often deterrents to international reporting. Through the use of the informal network, it was possible to alert the official sector of the suspicion of an avian influenza outbreak among poultry, without jeopardizing the reporting individual. The official report of an avian influenza outbreak ongoing in Indonesia was made to the OIE on 4 February 2004 [17]. In this instance there was a time lag of 3 months between the informal sector notification of a suspected outbreak and the formal sector notification.

A similar time lag was seen with the early reports of suspected avian influenza in Thailand. On 5 January 2004, the following was posted on ProMED-mail:

AVIAN INFLUENZA – THAILAND: RFI
****

Date: Sun, 5 Jan 2004
From: ProMED-mail <promed@promedmail.org>
Source: Malaysia Star, 5 Jan 2004 [edited]
<http://www.thestar.com.my/news/story.asp?file=2004/1/5/nation/7036583&sec=nation>

Penang farmers fear smuggled Thai chicks may spread bird flu

The Penang Poultry Farmers Association has voiced concerns about the possibility of live chicken smuggled from Thailand being infected with the bird flu...a report yesterday that the Terengganu Livestock Breeders Association had urged the state Veterinary Services Department to control the entry of chicken from Thailand following the detection of a virus that causes avian influenza among birds in that country [18].

The Thailand Department of Livestock refuted the above report on 9 January 2004, stating that the outbreak was due to fowl cholera, with the following caveat: "However, there might have been some confusion with an outbreak [in] mid-November 2003, of mixed infection of fowl cholera (*Pasteurella multocida* type A) and acute pasteurellosis (*Pasteurella haemolytica*) in one layer farm [of] about 68 000 birds at Nong Bua district in Nakorn Sawan province" [19].

In response to the early reports on suspected avian influenza in Thailand, the Thai Ministry of Health increased human influenza surveillance in provinces where there had been reports of major poultry die-offs. On 23 January 2004 there were simultaneous reports confirming avian influenza cases in the avian population, and in three humans [20, 21].

Again the sequence of events involved informal sector reports leading to formal sector reports at a later date (approximately 18 days). This demonstrates the importance of the communication of risk and the impact on heightening surveillance.

Similar time lags were also seen with reports of avian influenza in Vietnam.

2.3. CHIKUNGUNYA – INDIAN OCEAN

In May 2005, there was a posting on ProMED-mail describing an outbreak of Chikungunya in Mauritius and Reunion Island:

CHIKUNGUNYA – MAURITIUS AND REUNION ISLAND
****
Date: Wed, May 18, 2005
From: Mohammad Issack

In Mauritius, since early April 2005, several people have been attending the hospital and health centres of the capital city, Port-Louis, with fever and arthralgia of hands and feet... a rash was also noted.

Chikungunya virus was suspected based on the clinical presentation, the self-limiting course, and the recent report on ProMED-mail of a Chikungunya virus disease epidemic in the Comoros Islands [22].

The reporting physician was an astute clinician who had heard of Chikungunya virus activity in a neighboring island; he decided to send specimens for testing to determine whether a new outbreak in his area might be related. He also mentioned that the first cases in Mauritius occurred near a hostel where many students from the Comoros Islands were lodging [22].

2.4.   CLOSTRIDIUM NOVYI – INJECTING DRUG USERS UNITED KINGDOM

Injecting drug users frequently present to hospital emergency rooms with overwhelming sepsis, a condition associated with high mortality rates. Because of this, hospital personnel do not generally report these deaths to the official health sector as unusual events. In May 2000, ProMED-mail received the following report from an academic veterinarian at the Norwegian Army Medical School:

> ANTHRAX, HUMAN – NORWAY: RFI
> ************************************
> Date: 6 May 2000
> From: Per Lausund
>
> The press (Norwegian Broadcasting Corp.) has reported that a drug addict (IV heroin) died some days ago from anthrax. It is reported that the heroin might have been the source of the bacteria, but at the same time they warn drug abusers to watch out for sores with black crusts and scabs. This sounds like cutaneous anthrax. ...On the other hand, no more deaths or infections have been reported, and if this was in the drug abusers' heroin it should affect more than one person.
>
> Anyone heard of similar cases recently? [23]

Based on this report, there was an international alert regarding the possibility of anthrax contaminated heroin, which could constitute intentional introduction of a biologic agent. During this heightened alert, reports began to surface of an increase in deaths among injecting drug users in the UK. On 11 May 2000 there was a newswire report of eight unexplained deaths among injecting drug users in Scotland [24].

By 15 June 2000 there had been reports of 42 cases in Scotland and 20 cases in England and Wales. A diagnosis of disease due to infection with *Clostridium novyi* was made [25]. Full descriptions of the outbreaks were detailed in the literature, with mention that the initial alert was related to the case of anthrax in the injecting drug user in Norway [26, 27]. A total of 26 cases in England and 82 cases in Scotland and Ireland were identified as related to this outbreak. Retrospective active case finding did identify cases prior to April 2000, further supporting the observation that the heightened alert for adverse health events among injecting drug users, triggered by the anthrax case in Norway, led to the identification of this outbreak.

3.   Lessons Learned

The key lessons learned from the outbreak investigations detailed above are:

1.   We live in a global village where microbial organisms do not need visas for international travel.

2. No single institution has the capacity to address all needs and cover all bases with respect to disease surveillance.
3. Early alerts are important in preventing rumors and speculation, and in alerting the "astute clinicians" elsewhere to look for possible new problems in their areas.

In the event of an intentional biologic event, a communication of the risk (a disease process or outbreak) will lead to earlier suspicion of the same problem in other geographic areas. In the case of intentional release of a biologic agent, the scope of geographic involvement is not initially known; alerting the community quickly, especially the health-care community is a critical step in enhancing surveillance.

There is consensus that no one organization alone can cover all disease surveillance needs; a network of networks is necessary.

Informal sector reports can lead to formal sector investigations, resulting in earlier identification of emerging infectious diseases. This is especially true when dealing with new diseases (such as Nipah virus and SARS) or in the identification of known diseases in new geographic areas (such as Rift Valley fever on the Arabian peninsula, and West Nile virus infections in the Americas).

4.   Conclusions

The case studies of outbreak reports presented above serve to underscore the important role the informal sector plays in providing early warnings of disease risks. ProMED-mail is a good example of drawing upon the resources of the informal sector, through a listserv that broadcasts alerts of potential health risks based on reports from individual subscribers and those found in the lay press. This electronic means of communication of potential health risks has been successful as an early warning system for emerging diseases to both the formal health sector as well as the community at large. It further demonstrates that multiple-disease-reporting systems are complementary and enhance the early detection of unusual health events.

The role of the astute clinician cannot be understated. In the event of the intentional release of a biologic agent, early communication of the risk would assist the astute clinician in early recognition of a problem in his or her community.

Acknowledgments

Editorial assistance and guidance from Paul Guttry and Isaac Druker is very much appreciated. The ProMED-mail Editor, Associate Editors, and

Moderators must be recognized for their contributions leading to the actual postings on the ProMED-mail service: Lawrence Madoff, Stuart Handysides, Donald Kaye, Jack Woodall, Peter Cowen, J. Allan Dodds, Tam Garland, Martin Hughes-Jones, Larry Lutwick, Eskild Petersen, Craig Pringle, Michael Service, Arnon Shimshony, and Tom Yuill.

References

1. Madoff LC. ProMED-mail: an early warning system for emerging diseases. CID 2004:39 (15 July) 227–232.
2. Woodall JP. Global surveillance of emerging diseases: the ProMED-mail perspective. Cad. Saúde Pública 2001; 17(Suppl.).
3. Australian Government Department of Health and Aging Australia's notifiable diseases status, 2000: Annual report of the National Notifiable Diseases Surveillance System, Communicable Diseases Intelligence, June 2000; 26(2). Available at: http://www.health.gov.au/internet/wcms/Publishing.nsf/Content/cda-pubs-cdi-2002-cdi2602-cdi2602b6.htm. Accessed 2 January 2007.
4. Cleaveland S, Laurenson MK, Taylor LH. Diseases of humans and their domestic mammals: pathogen characteristics, host range and the risk of emergence. Philos Trans R Soc Lond B Biol Sci 2001; 356:991–999.
5. ProMED-mail. Pneumonia–China (Guangdong): RFI. ProMED-mail archive 20030210.0357. 10 February 2003. Available at: http://www.promedmail.org. Accessed 5 June 2005.
6. World Health Organization, Summary of probable SARS cases with onset of illness from 1 November 2002–31 July 2003 (Based on data as of 31 December 2003). Available at: http://www.who.int/csr/sars/country/table2004_04_21/en/index.html. Accessed 3 January 2007.
7. ProMED-mail. Undiagnosed illness–Vietnam (Hanoi): RFI. ProMEDmail archive 20030311.0595. 11 March 2003. Available at: http://www.promedmail.org. Accessed 5 June 2005.
8. Poutanen SM, Low DE, Henry B, et al. Identification of severe acute respiratory syndrome in Canada. N Engl J Med 2003; 348:1995–2005.
9. Webster RG, Bean WJ, Gorman OT, Chambers TM, Kawaoka Y. Evolution and ecology of influenza A viruses. Microbiol Mol Biol Rev 1992 March; 56(1): 152–179.
10. ProMED-mail. Influenza, bird-to-man, first case? ProMED-mail archive 19970820.1747. 20 August 1997. Available at: http://www.promedmail.org. Accessed 7 January 2007.
11. ProMED-mail. Influenza, bird-to-man, first case? (02). ProMED-mail archive 19970821.1750. 21 August 1997. Available at: http://www.promedmail.org. Accessed 7 January 2007.
12. ProMED-mail. Influenza, bird-to-man, - China (Hong Kong) (12). ProMED-mail archive 19971209.2452. 9 December 1997. Available at: http://www.promedmail.org. Accessed 7 January 2007.

13. ProMED-mail. Influenza, H5N1 human case – China (Hong Kong). ProMED-mail archive 20030219.0428. 19 February 2003. Available at: http://www.promedmail.org. Accessed 7 January 2007.

14. Sims LD et al. Origin and evolution of highly pathogenic H5N1 avian influenza in Asia. Vet Rec 2005; 157:159.

15. ProMED-mail. Influenza, bird-to-man, first case? (04). Archive 19970825.1766. 25 August 1007. Available at: http://www.promedmail.org. Accessed 7 January 2007.

16. ProMED-mail. Avian influenza – Indonesia: RFI. Archive 20031119.2872. 19 November 2003. Available at: http://www.promedmail.org. Accessed 5 June 2005.

17. ProMED-mail. Avian influenza – Indonesia: OIE Archive 20040204.0413. 4 February 2004. Available at: http://www.promedmail.org. Accessed 5 June 2005. Based on a published report by OIE at a URL no longer accessible.(http://www.oie.int/Messages/040203IDN.htm)

18. ProMED-mail. Avian influenza – Thailand: RFI. Archive 20040105.0051. 5 January 2004. Available at: http://www.promedmail.org. Accessed 5 June 2005.

19. ProMED-mail. Avian influenza – Thailand (02): not confirmed. Archive 20040109.0097. 9 January 2004. Available at: http://www.promedmail.org. Accessed 5 June 2005.

20. ProMED-mail. Avian influenza, Thailand – OIE. Archive 20040124.0276. 24 January 2004. Available at: http://www.promedmail.org. Accessed 5 June 2005.

21. ProMED-mail. Avian influenza, human – Thailand (02): confirmed. Archive 20040123.0262. 23 January 2004. Available at: http://www.promedmail.org. Accessed 5 June 2005.

22. ProMED-mail. Chikungunya – Mauritius and Reunion Island. Archive 20050519.1372. 19 May 2005. Available at: http://www.promedmail.org. Accessed 5 June 2005.

23. ProMED-mail. Anthrax, human – Norway: RFI. Archive 20000506.0119. 6 May 2000. Available at: http://www.promedmail.org. Accessed 5 June 2005.

24. ProMED-mail. Unexplained deaths, human – UK (Scotland). Archive 20000511.0717. 11 May 2000. Available at: http://www.promedmail.org. Accessed 5 June 2005.

25. ProMED-mail. Unexplained deaths, drug addicts – UK: diagnosis. 20000615.0977. 15 June 2000. Available at: http://www.promedmail.org. Accessed 5 June 2005.

26. Jones JA., et al. An outbreak of serious illness and death among injecting drug users in England during 2000. J Med Microbiol 2002; 51: 978–984.

27. Fischer MA. An outbreak of histiotoxic clostridial infections among injection drug users in Scotland and Ireland. Presented at the Intersci Conf Antimicrob Agents Chemother Intersci Conf Antimicrob Agents Chemother 2001 Dec 16–19; 41: abstract no. 2009. Meeting abstract available at: http://gateway.nlm.nih.gov/MeetingAbstracts/102270101.html. Accessed 7 January 2007.

INFORMATION SYSTEMS FOR RISK COMMUNICATION RELATED TO BIOTERRORISM

Manfred S. Green[1,2] and Zalman Kaufman[1]

[1]Israel Center for Disease Control, Ministry of Health, Tel Hashomer, Israel and [2]Faculty of Medicine, Tel Aviv University, Israel

1.   Abstract

The goal of bioterrorism is to create panic in the population and disrupt the society. Risk communication can play a pivotal role in mitigating the effects of a bioterrorist event. Since the perception of risk is frequently no less important than the actual risk, the availability of reliable, credible, and timely information can be critical for effective risk communication. For this purpose, new data sources and the means of utilizing them need to be developed. In this chapter, we discuss the role of information systems in risk communication and provide examples of the type of data needed at the different stages of a bioterrorist event.

2.   Introduction

In his report to Congress in November 2001, Kenneth Shine, then president of the National Institute of Medicine, defined the goal of the terrorist as "an attempt to produce fear, magnified by an exaggerated sense of risk .... and perpetuated by misinformation and rumors" [1]. Bioterrorism has characteristics which make it particularly "attractive" to achieve these goals, since it can dramatically increase the fear of impending disease and death in the entire population. In addition, the uncertainty surrounding a bioterror incident can generate fertile soil for sowing the seeds of mistrust in the ability of the authorities to control the incident. This mistrust is a guaranteed recipe for generating public panic, with resultant adverse effects on the public services and the economy. Examples of panic caused by bioterrorism or chemical terrorism include the deliberate salmonella outbreak in the United States [2], the deliberate use of sarin gas in Japan [3] and the distribution of anthrax spores through the mail in the United States [4].

M.S. Green et al. (eds.), Risk Assessment and Risk Communication Strategies in Bioterrorism Preparedness, 177–191.

In order to reduce the impact of a bioterrorism event, risk management strategies should be implemented. These includes mitigation strategies that are geared toward both decreasing the impact of a future risk and coping strategies that are intended to relieve the impact once the risk (the event) has occurred [5]. Risk communication plays a major role in both these components. In order to be effective, risk communication should be based on solid data and should be informative, understandable, consistent, accurate, complete, and timely. In this chapter, we discuss the role of information in developing effective risk communication in the event of a bioterrorist attack. This will be examined in terms of the public perception of risk and what are termed "acceptable" and "unacceptable" risks.

3.   Public Perception of Risk

Both the type of information related to the risk and the way it is conveyed will influence the public's perception of risk. The expert's approach has been contrasted with the layperson's perspective of risk [6–8]. It has been suggested that while the expert asks objective questions, such as whether there is a potential risk, what is its nature, what dose will induce a harmful effect and how significant is the risk, the layperson may find risk statistics either less important or they may take on different meanings. For example, risk may be perceived by the layperson in the framework of routine events, heavily influenced by the media. Others suggested that public reactions to risk often have a rationality of their own and proposed that "expert" and "lay" perspectives should inform each other as part of a two-way process [9]. From either perspective, the availability of good data will influence both the expert and the layman in judging the seriousness of the risk and whether it can be contained.

4.   Acceptable and Unacceptable Risks

The type of risk is also an important consideration in the public's perception of risk. Fischhoff et al. [10] delineate the term they referred to as "acceptable risks". These are generally voluntary risks, risks under an individual's control, risks with clear benefits, risks fairly distributed, risks generated by a trusted source, and risks perceived to be familiar. In contrast he described less acceptable risks as those that are, in general, "involuntary, inequitably distributed, inescapable by taking personal precautions, arise from an unfamiliar or novel source, result from man-made, rather than natural sources, cause hidden and irreversible damage and poorly understood by science" [9]. The risk of bioterrorism would clearly fall in the latter category. The fact that the risk may be perceived as being associated with hidden and irreversible damage and poorly understood by science needs to be countered with the best data available.

5.   Risk Communication

The overall goals of risk communication are to minimize panic and encourage rational behavior thus helping to minimize morbidity, mortality, and the impact on the social and economic infrastructure. Risk communication has been described as: "the interactive exchange of information and opinions throughout the risk analysis process ... including the explanation of risk assessment findings and the basis of risk management decisions" [11]. Among the seven "cardinal rules of risk communication" Covello and Allen [12] proposed "accepting and involving the public as a partner, listening to the public's specific concerns, working with other credible sources and meeting the needs of the media". Chess et al. [13] stressed the need to interact with the community, identify, and respond to the needs of different audiences and recognize that people's values and feelings are a legitimate aspect of health issues. In such circumstances, the availability of reliable, timely, and constantly updated data can help put the risk in a clearer perspective. These data can also be used to help predict the course of events and address the so-called "What if ....?" factor, described by Langford et al. [14]. They suggested that the risk communicators should "ensure that there is a "safety net" of protection, should reasonable safety procedures be found inadequate and indicate beforehand how such arrangements will be put in place and be made accessible." Such reassurances should be backed up by good data.

6.   Stages in Risk Communication Associated with a Bioterrorist Event

As a convenient conceptual and operative framework, risk communication associated with a bioterrorist event may be divided into five stages, according to the need for data at each stage. The first stage is prior to the event, the second on suspicion of an event, the third on confirmation of the event, the fourth during the event, and the fifth following the event. At each stage, the public is likely to ask questions relevant to that stage. The main questions that are likely to be raised prior to a bioterrorist incident are whether in fact it can occur, and are the authorities well-prepared for the possibility. The main question on suspicion of an event is whether we are witnessing the first stages of a bioterrorist incident. The questions on confirmation of an incident include: where is it located, when did it start, is it contagious, am I at risk, and is there a cure? The questions during the event include: is the treatment effective, is the disease spreading, am I at risk, and when will it end? The questions after the event focus on whether the event has really ended and is there still a risk of exposure. The ability of the authorities to respond adequately to these questions depends on their access to good data on which to base their answers.

7.   Sources of Data for Risk Communication

The sources of information for risk communication will depend on the stage of the incident. Prior to the confirmed incident, a system which monitors usual morbidity patterns and assesses the possibilities of anomalies is important. Syndromic-type surveillance is typically based on initial nonspecific signs and symptoms in patients visiting primary care physicians or emergency rooms. It is used as a crude, but early and timely monitoring of the incidence rates of infectious diseases prior to definitive diagnoses. On suspicion of an event, syndromic surveillance data could be used to rapidly evaluate whether there is unusual morbidity related either or both in time and place to the suspected cases. In the third stage, on confirmation of one or more cases, several data sources would be used to determine the current extent of the outbreak. These would include syndromic surveillance data, hospitalization admissions with presenting complaints, information on requests for blood cultures and confirmed isolates. In the fourth stage, during the outbreak, syndromic type data together with confirmed diagnoses could be used to determine the extent of both the size and geographical distribution of the outbreak. In the fifth stage, at the end of the outbreak, syndromic surveillance could be used to respond to rumors of continuation of the outbreak or signs of a new outbreak. In all situations, analytic methods such as time series analysis, geographical information system (GIS), and cluster analysis are helpful aids for evaluating and presenting the data.

Theoretical examples of the kind of data that may be useful during the five stages of a bioterrorist incident are shown in Figures 1–4. Three types of data are shown. Figures 1a, b show the presentation of a suspicious event which is ruled out when examined in the perspective of historical syndromic surveillance data. In the third and fourth stage, Figures 2a–c show graphical presentation of syndromic type data demonstrating the emergence of an anomaly in a particular area compared with historical background of morbidity and morbidity in the rest of the country. In addition, for the third and fourth stages, Figure 3 presents the results of analyses using GIS to map in more detail the geographical distribution of the suspected cases. At all stages, Figures 4a–c show the actual and predicted epidemic curves use to track the progress of the epidemic based on both suspected cases (including those based on syndromic surveillance) and confirmed cases.

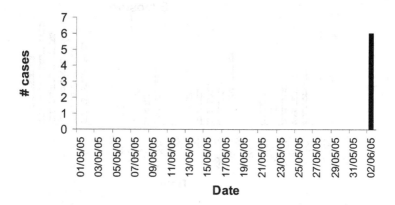

Figure 1a. Six patients admitted to an ER in Tel Aviv, suffering from pneumonia. Is it unusual?

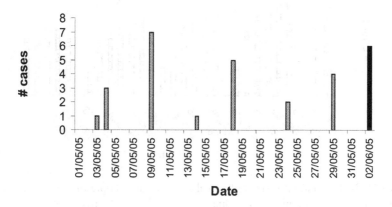

Figure 1b. Compare current with past morbidity, based on syndromic surveillance data.

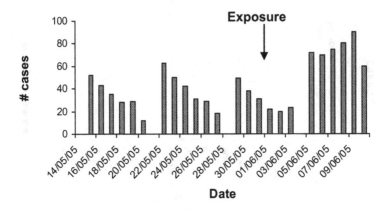

Figure 2a. Visits to community clinics in Tel Aviv due to influenza-like illness, based on syndromic surveillance data.

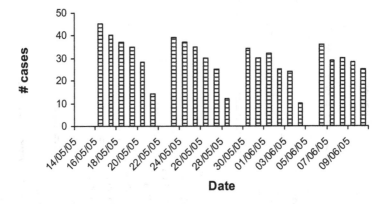

Figure 2b. Is the incident restricted to Tel Aviv, or are people in other areas also at risk? Visits to community clinics due to flu-like illness at a neighboring city.

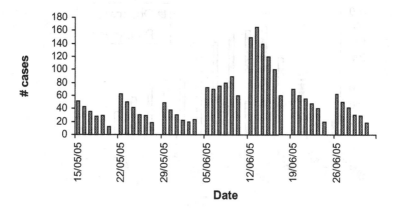

Figure 2c. Visits to community clinic due to flu-like Illness returned to baseline.

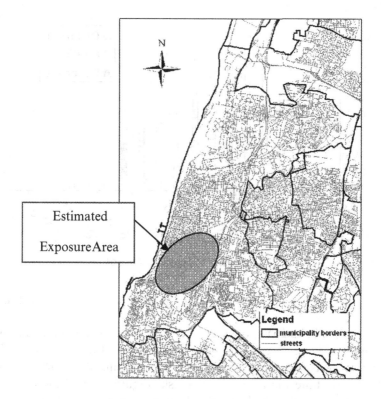

Figure 3. What is the exposed area?

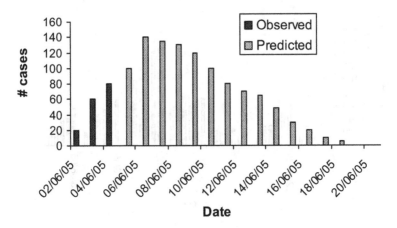

Figure 4a. How many people have become ill and when will it end? Predictor models.

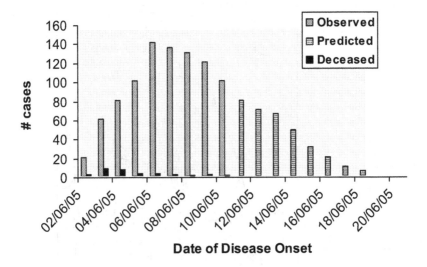

Figure 4b. How many people have been diagnosed until now and when it will end?

Figure 1 could be the basis of assurance to the public that nothing unusual has occurred. Figure 2 could provide nonspecific data, suggesting the beginning of an event. Figure 3 is useful for mapping the distribution of cases to demonstrate the areas of high risk. Figure 4 show the evolving epidemic curves based on both specific diagnoses and suspected cases based on nonspecific signs and symptoms. At each stage, the epidemic curve could be used both to predict the progression of the outbreak and demonstrate

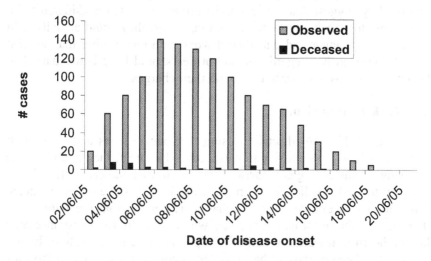

Figure 4c. No additional new cases originating from the incident.

the decline and end of the outbreak. The figures show both what is likely to be seen at each stage and what the real picture will be at the end of the incident.

8.   Myths in Risk Communication and The Role of Information

There are frequently misconceptions about what information should and should not be presented to the public. In this regard, Chess et al. [13] described some myths in risk communication and suggested ways to deal with them. This demonstrates the need for availability of good data at all stages in order to respond to them. They also suggested that the myth that we should not go to the public until we have solutions should actually be countered by the action to release and discuss information about risk [13]. This clearly implies that the authorities have access to reliable information and stresses the need for ongoing comprehensive data collection. Furthermore, Chess et al. contend that the myth that telling the public about a risk is more likely to unduly alarm could be countered by the argument that you can decrease potential for alarm by giving people a chance to express their concerns. In this regard, we need to ask whether we have adequate data on which to base our answers?

A common myth they describe is that the issues are too difficult for the public to understand. In this situation, the availability of good data can be extremely useful for conveying comprehensible messages to the public.

Finally, they suggest that while activist groups are often considered to be responsible for stirring up unwarranted concerns, they could actually help to focus public anger and one should work with them rather than against them. Clearly, in this regard, the authorities should have better data than the activist groups in order to cope with their charges.

9.   Risk Comparisons

Covello et al. [15, 16] discussed using risk comparisons and stated that comparisons can help put risk in perspective. However, they point out that irrelevant or misleading comparisons can harm trust and credibility. Thus, in order to make valid risk comparisons, it is assumed that adequate information is available. One also has to remember that the public will often believe that information is being withheld. A frequent response may then be hostility toward the authorities, perhaps due to frustration. In any event, it has been proposed that in order to emphasize that the authorities are in control, it is a mistake to pretend that the risk is minimal or nonexistent [17]. Good data sources could be used to present a realistic evaluation of the risk.

10.   Dealing with Overreaction

Taig [18] has discussed the problem of overreaction or panic when new information about risk is made public and the difficulty in rejecting ineffective and expensive solutions that have captured the public imagination. Once again, availability of good data is important for gaining public trust. Proposed ineffective solutions can only be rejected if they can be evaluated in the light of good data. In specifically relating to risk communication to a bioterrorism incident, Sandman [19] has proposed that one should not "over-reassure, acknowledge uncertainty and share dilemmas". He suggested that one should "acknowledge and legitimate people's fears". Clearly, good data can help to put these fears in perspective. For example, answers to the "what-if" questions should be backed up by data.

11.   Dealing with the Media

Availability of reliable data is critical for developing an atmosphere of trust between the authorities and the media. Advice on how to deal with media has been proposed by Donovan and Covello [20]. The suggestions were to speak only on what you know, say that you do not know and offer to get the information by a specified time. This assumes that you have access to additional data. When giving reasons why you cannot answer, the public should know that you are actively collecting good and comprehensive data. Responses to rumors can be much more effective if they are based on the availability of good data.

12.   Example of Risk Communication During the United States Anthrax Incident

The anthrax incident in the United States in 2001 [4] provides a good example of the data issues when the authorities dealt with risk communication at the different stages described above. During stage 1, about 2 months prior to the incident, the authorities issued statements to prepare the population for the possibility for a bioterrorist attack. For example, on August 16, 2001, the Department of Health and Human Services issued a Press Release as follows: "While the exact risks are unknown .... the use of biological weapons by terrorists, potentially could result in life-threatening illness on a large scale. Even a lone terrorist could cause a major outbreak in the population" [21]. At this stage, the public would want to know what mechanisms are in place for monitoring for unusual disease activity and what data are available to the authorities. Routine syndromic-type surveillance could be used as an example in this area.

During stage 2, suspicion of a possible bioterrorist event was raised when a case of inhalational anthrax was diagnosed in Florida on October 4, 2001. The media was informed the following day by United States Health and Human Services Secretary, Tommy Thompson, that: "An isolated case of anthrax infection was confirmed on Thursday in a Florida hospital. There is no evidence of terrorism. The man could have picked up the infection from his clothes and was known to have drunk water from a creek recently" [22]. Later, on October 4, the Centers for Disease Control and Prevention (CDC) issued a press release: "The last case of anthrax was in Texas earlier this year. No need for the public to take extraordinary steps. No need to buy and horde medicines or antibiotics." [23]. In fact, the case in Texas earlier that year was not inhalation anthrax, and the information was incomplete. At this stage, it could have been useful to have active monitoring of syndromic surveillance type data to back up the impression that nothing unusual had yet occurred. This would provide data for risk communication.

Stage 3 began with a real suspicion of a possible bioterrorist event, when on October 9, the press reported that a second case had been detected in a colleague of the first case. Nevertheless, they reported that experts cautioned against jumping to conclusions without backing up this statement with any data [24]. Asked whether this could be related to bioterrorism, a spokesman for the Florida Department of Health said: "This would take a turn in our investigation. We were thinking more of environmental sources" [24]. The public's confidence could have been bolstered by being told that a monitoring system was in place and examples of the type of temporal and spatial data being collected could be presented.

On October 11, the CDC issued a press release as follows: "CDC is far enough in this investigation to reassure the public that this appears to be a local and isolated exposure focused in one building. Nevertheless, CDC is not packing up and going home" [25]. By October 16, there was recognition of the fact that this was likely to be a bioterrorist attack, and thus moved into stage 3. The CDC issued a press release in which they cautioned that "there may be more reports of cases. This is the disease monitoring system in action. The system is working" [26]. The question here is what monitoring system is working. The public need more detailed information on the system and what information it can provide.

On October 23, in a press release by the Health and Human Services (HHS), Secretary of Health Tommy Thompson reassured Americans that "they should continue to live their lives with confidence". "He stated that "America's citizens can be sure that their government agencies are ready to respond to biological warfare and bioterrorism quickly and effectively throughout the country" [27]. Once again, the public needs to know how the situation is being monitored, including the uncertainties, so as to be able to cope with surprises.

Stage 5 was late in the course of events, and Dr. Jeffrey Koplan, Director of the CDC, in a telebriefing on October 25 said: "People are surprised that we're learning things on a day-by-day basis. You always wish that you knew on day one, what you know on day 20" [25]. The public could reasonably ask what is it that you know on day 20 that you would have liked to know on day 1, and why that information was not available.

Stage 5 was also evident on October 17, essentially at the end of the incident, when the Mail Service issued a press release stating that "The mail is safe. People shouldn't stop using the mail because of these isolated incidents. We have delivered more than 2 billion items since Sept 11. Pay attention to incoming mail. Everyone should exercise common sense" [28]. Once again, the public needs to know what data were available on which to base this recommendation and what kind of monitoring is in place.

13.   Public Information Sources for Risk Communication

In the aftermath of the incident, during stage 5, the president of the National Institute of Medicine, in a report to Congress on November 29, 2001, discussed the question of information to the public. He cautioned the public to "seek authoritative information on anthrax from three web sites only ... because of our concern about the amount of misinformation being conveyed about the anthrax incidents ...and the confusion that had resulted from multiple sources of analysis, commentary and advice". In retrospect, a Gallup Poll on October 31, 2001, found that 43% believed that the government was providing the public with reliable information whereas 30% believed that the government itself lacked reliable information [29]. Thus, the fact that a large percentage of the public believed that the government did not have access to adequate information creates a situation of suspicion and mistrust, a possible basis for panic responses.

Ethical issues on risk communication need to be addressed. For example, what information should be supplied to the public and what information does the public want? Who should supply this information and in what detail? To what extent should information be withheld in order to avoid panic?

14.   Conclusions

Availability of good data helps the authorities to provide information to the public which puts the incident and its associated risks in the correct perspective. It also engenders confidence that the authorities are taking well-informed decisions.

References

1. Kenneth Shine, For a hearing on risk communication: national security and public health (testimony presented to the Subcommittee on National Security, Veterans Affairs, and International Relations, House Committee on Government Reform, Washington, DC: 29 Nov., 2001). Available at: www7.nationalacademies.org/ocga/testimony/Risk_Communication_Natl_ Security_Public_Health.asp. Accessed 4 July 2006.
2. Torok T, Tauxe RV, Wise RP, et al. A large community outbreak of Salmonella caused by intentional contamination of restaurant salad bars. JAMA 1997; 278:389–395.

3. Ohtani T, Iwanami A, Kasai K, Yamasue H, Kato T, Sasaki T, Kato N. Post-traumatic stress disorder symptoms in victims of Tokyo subway attack: a 5-year follow-up study. Psychiatry Clin Neurosci 2004; 58:624–629.

4. Maillard J-M, Fischer M, McKee KT Jr., Turner LF, Cline JS. First case of bioterrorism-related inhalational anthrax, Florida, 2001: North Carolina Investigation. Emerg Infect Dis 2002; 8:1035–1038.

5. Department for Environment, Food and Rural Affairs, UK. Risk management strategy. Available at: www.defra.gov.uk/corporate/busplan/riskmanage/index.htm. Accessed 9 July 2006.

6. Mertz CK, Slovic P, Purchase IFH. Judgments of chemical risks: comparison among senior managers, toxicologists, and the public. Risk Analysis 1998; 18:391–404.

7. Slovic P. Perception of risk. Science 1987; 236:280–285.

8. Slovic P, Malmfors T, Krewski D, Mertz CK, Neil N, Bartlett S. Intuitive toxicology. II. Expert and lay judgments of chemical risks in Canada. Risk Analysis 1995; 15:661–675.

9. Bennett P. Understanding responses to risk: some basic findings. In: Bennett P and Calman K (ed.). Risk Communication of Public Health. Oxford: Oxford University Press, 1999.

10. Fischhoff B, Lichtenstein S, Slovic P, Keeney D. Acceptable risk. Cambridge, MA: Cambridge University Press, 1981.

11. Covello VT, Peters RG, Wojtecki JG, Hyde RC. Risk communication, the West Nile virus epidemic, and bioterrorism: responding to the communication challenges posed by the intentional or unintentional release of a pathogen in an urban setting. J Urban Health 2001; 78:382–391.

12. Covello V, Allen F. 1988. Seven cardinal rules of risk communication. US Environmental Protection Agency, Office of Policy Analysis, Washington, DC.

13. Chess C, Hance BJ, Sandman PM. improving dialogue with communities: a short guide to government risk communication. Trenton, NJ: Department of Environmental Protection, 1988.

14. Langford IH, Marris C, O'Riordan T. Public reactions to risks: social structures, images of science, and role of trust. In: Bennett P and Calman K (eds). Risk Communication and Public Health. Oxford: Oxford University Press, 1999. pp. 3–50.

15. Covello V. Issues and problems in using risk comparisons for communicating right-to-know information on chemical risks. Environ Sci Technol 1989; 23:1444–1449.

16. Covello V. (1998). Communicating risk information: a guide to environmental communication in crisis and non-crisis situations, with principles of effective risk communication in crisis and noncrisis situations. In: Kolluru RV (ed.). Environmental strategies handbook: a guide to effective policies and practices. New York: McGraw-Hill.

17. Agency for Toxic Substances and Disease Registry. A primer on health risk communication principles and practices. Available at: www.atsdr.cdc.gov/HEC/primer.html. Accessed 9 July 2006.

18. Taig T. Benchmarking in government: case studies and principles. In: Bennett P and Calman K (eds). Risk Communication and Public Health. Oxford: Oxford University Press, 1999. pp. 117–132.

19. Sandman PM. Bioterrorism risk communication policy. J Health Commun 2003; 8(Suppl 1):146–147; discussion 148–151.

20. Donovan E, Covello V. Risk communication student manual. Chemical Manufacturers' Association, Washington, DC, 1989.

21. United States Department of Health & Human Services. HHS initiative prepares for possible bioterrorism threat. Available at: www.hhs.gov/news/press/2001pres/01fsbioterrorism.html. Accessed 14 May 2006.

22. Harnden T, Fenton B. Pleas for calm in Florida as Briton catches anthrax. Published in the Telegraph web site on 05/10/2001. Available at: www.telegraph.co.uk/news/main.jhtml?xml=/news/2001/10/05/wanth05.xml. Accessed 14 May 2006.

23. Centers for Disease Control and Prevention. Press release on 4 October 2001: public health message regarding anthrax case. Available at: www.cdc.gov/od/oc/media/pressrel/r011004.htm. Accessed 14 May 2006.

24. Online News Hour. Second anthrax case reported in Florida. Available at: www.pbs.org/newshour/updates/october01/anthrax_10-8.html. Accessed 4 July 2006.

25. Centers for Disease Control and prevention. Anthrax update: 25 October 2001, telebriefing transcript. Available at: www.cdc.gov/od/oc/media/transcripts/t011025.html. Accessed 4 July 2006.

26. Centers for Disease Control and prevention. Press release on 16 October 2001: update: anthrax investigations, Florida and New York. Available at: www.cdc.gov/od/oc/media/pressrel/r011016.htm Accessed 14 May 2006.

27. United States Department of Health & Human Services. Secretary Thompson testifies on HHS readiness and role of vaccine research and development. Available at: www.hhs.gov/news/pree/2001pres/20011023.html. Accessed 14 May 2006.

28. United States Postal Service. USPS message to customers: we are taking every possible measure to assure safety of customers and the mail, 17 October 2001. Available at: www.usps.com/news/2001/press/pr01_1010tips.htm. Accessed 4 July 2006.

29. Public would rather have vague terror warnings than none at all. Public Agenda Special Edition: Terrorism. Updated 7 November 2001. Available at: www.publicagenda.org/specials/terrorism/110701terror_pubopinion.htm. Accessed 4 July 2006.

Part III

FOCUS ON SMALLPOX

RISK ASSESSMENT IN SMALLPOX BIOTERRORIST AGGRESSION

Marian Negut

National Institute of R&D for Microbiology & Immunology Cantacuzino, Bucharest, Romania

1. Abstract

As many specialists pointed out, a bioterrorist attack using a smallpox virus becomes an increasing probability. Global susceptibility of the population, high transmissibility, lack of specific treatment, difficult and late clinical diagnosis of first cases, and impressive and severe clinical pictures are important factors of risk assessment in smallpox terrorist aggression.

Airborne, the major way of spreading, intensive and long-distance traveling, and absence of bioprevention measures increase dramatically the epidemic extension. Under these circumstances, the capacity to limit aggression is rapidly overcome. So, risk assessment is one of the most important steps of bioprevention strategy of smallpox aggression.

2. Introduction

"The September 11, 2001 attacks on the World Trade Center and Pentagon changed forever our collective thinking with regard to our vulnerability to terrorist attacks" [7]. Less than one month later on October 4, 2003, a criminal anthrax epidemic lasting almost two months demonstrated the reality of large impact of present-day bioterrorism. Several scenarios were imagined on the possible future bioterrorist attacks. Among potential agents variola virus was estimated as one of the most probably used [2, 5, 7].

2.1. SMALLPOX: A FORGOTTEN DISEASE?

In 1980, World Health Organization (WHO) certified smallpox eradication worldwide and officially variola virus storage was restricted to two WHO reference laboratories: the Center for Disease Control and Prevention (CDC) in Atlanta, USA and State Research Center for Virology and Biotechnology "Vector" at Koltsovo, in Novosibirsk, Russia. All other

M.S. Green et al. (eds.), Risk Assessment and Risk Communication Strategies in Bioterrorism Preparedness, 195–203.

laboratories in the world were required to destroy their remaining variola virus stocks. In 1996, WHO General Assembly decided to destroy the stocks in 1999. But in 1999, the destruction was postponed until 2002. An advisory Committee of variola virus research proposed a program of work and indefinite postponement was admitted, so nowadays live smallpox virus stocks exist officially [16]. Immense stockpiles of variola virus were held by former Soviet Union at Sergiev Posad; the secret plant, as Dr. Alibek said, still exists and by Dr. Henderson's opinion remains as a focus of concern [9]. The black market trade in weapons of mass destruction is probably the only way of acquiring the virus. But this possibility exists and bioterrorism has no logic limits.

2.2.   WHY SMALLPOX?

According to the specialists, smallpox is a "very potential bioterrorism choice" as:

1. At present, there is a high and global receptivity to variola virus. After eradication and more than 30 years no vaccination was performed and average protection postvaccination is about 5–7 years. A stock of 200 million doses of prepared vaccine was saved for use in case of accidental outbreak. In the last 5 years many countries prepared necessary stockpile of vaccine against smallpox. But WHO does not recommend vaccination of individuals before the smallpox epidemic occurs because of side effects. Vaccinia immune globulin recommended for the treatment of serious side effects is in very limited quantity so that stockpiles of this globulin were suggested to be made along with smallpox vaccine [6].
2. Contagiousness of smallpox is higher than 80%. The first generation of cases would rapidly spread in highly susceptible population, expanding each generation of cases, by a factor of 10 times or more during winter or spring [9]. As was recently demonstrated by pandemic spreading of severe acute respiratory syndrome (SARS), this rapid extension of smallpox could be a global disaster. Long-distance traveling of un-detected human sources could represent the major way of pandemic spreading of smallpox also.
3. Clinical picture of smallpox has always had strong psychological impact in "civilian population", so this impact is expected to happen. Because of lack of immunoprotection a high proportion of severe clinical pictures involving long hospitalization is estimated. Unpredictable medical difficulties will be arised by the incapacity of medical authorities to cover these huge requirements. Mild cases will be home-isolated increasing epidemic risk and spreading [14, 15].

4. There is no specific antiviral treatment for smallpox. Thiosemicarbazones and rifampicin previously reported having therapeutic benefits proved to be ineffective [9]. Cidofivir, a nucleotide analog of DNA polymerase inhibitor, experimented in cytomegalovirus infection treatment suggested to be used in postexposure treatment rather for treatment of the diagnosed smallpox [9, 11].

5. The reported mortality of the smallpox was higher than 30%. Hemorrhagic and malignant forms are uniformly fatal [9, 14].

6. A violent psychosocial reaction is likely to appear at the beginning of the epidemic "smallpox fear." This psychological impact is more stronger in the population than in some other severe transmissible diseases.

Medical (clinical) impressive aspects, antiepidemic restrictive measures, current difficulties, and social perturbances could determine a psychosocial crisis followed by a real civilian panic [13].

3. Risk Assessment in Smallpox Bioaggression

The main areas of risk in smallpox bioaggression are presented in Figure 1. All these areas are influencing in between them in realizing very strong psychosocial perturbances that could degenerate in a strong panic of civilian population.

It is well known that one of the main targets of bioterrorist attack is to produce impressive psychosocial effects followed by socioeconomic perturbances and social disorganization.

This psychosocial impact influences in many aspects of clinical and epidemic side effects by magnifying difficulties of medical and antiepidemic intervention [13].

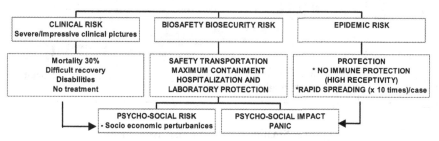

Figure 1. Risk areas in smallpox bioaggression.

3.1.   CLINICAL RISK ASSESSMENT

Clinical risk assessment is considered to be important. During the progression of the disease it has to take into account the following gravity factors in risk evaluation [5, 9, 14].

- Smallpox is an exclusively human disease and nowadays any case is an alleged manipulation of variola virus.
- The illness is expected to be very severe in the majority of cases as the population under 40 years has no variola, "immunologic specific memory" (the vaccination was stopped in many countries before 1977).
- There is no etiologic treatment in smallpox. So the hospitalization will be of long duration overcoming hospital capacities in an epidemic situation.
- Severe malignant and hemorrhagic forms are fatal always so mortality is overcoming 30% in smallpox. Immunodeficient patients, pregnancy, and chronic cardiac diseases are predisposing conditions to severe forms.
- Clinical recognition of the illness is difficult in the first stage in the absence of epidemic information/suspicion. First cases will have high epidemic potential.
- Laboratory confirmation is also late in the first cases because routine laboratory investigation does not include such a potential etiology.

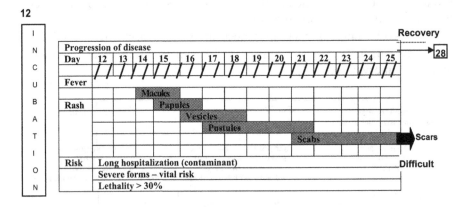

Figure 2. Smallpox – clinical risk assessment.

Figure 2 shows the risk during the progression of disease. Starting from the 10th day after contamination, the patient represents an important source of infection by respiratory droplets and later by the content of vesicles and pustules and at the end by scabs. The hospitalization in smallpox is compulsory in all the period of contagiousness that means minimum 3–4 weeks. In epidemic situation hospital capacities are overcome.

As the febrile onset is not specific, clinical presumption is late, when characteristic vesicles and pustules develop. In malignant forms, the diagnostic confusion is more frequent so first cases in absence of epidemic suspicion are "sacrificed patients" [9].

Laboratory identification of the virus in oropharyngeal exudate is possible by modern techniques (electron microscopy, immunoenzymatic detection, and molecular techniques) in less than 24 hours. Routine laboratory investigation does not include variola virus detection without any particular requirement. The confirmation of the first cases is late when virus detection is recommended from vesicles content (5–7 days of the progression of the disease) [3, 15].

No antiviral treatment is efficient in smallpox. The progression of the disease depends on the capacity of response of the patient. The estimated severity of the disease determines important vital risk. The historical known mortality of 30% is expected to be higher in absence of immune specific background [9].

Clinical factor will contribute substantially to increase associated psychosocial risk. Socioeconomic perturbances will increase psychosocial impact leading to "psychological mass reaction." Risk assessment of psychosocial reaction is as well important as medical risk.

Epidemic risk assessment is dominated by the high capacity of spreading of the disease in modern opportunities of dissemination and lack of any immune protection [2, 10].

The interdependence of the particular epidemic factors in smallpox is presented schematically in Figure 3.

As global extension of SARS demonstrated recently, long-distance traveling nowadays represents a major risk activation of rapid spreading of high-risk respiratory diseases.

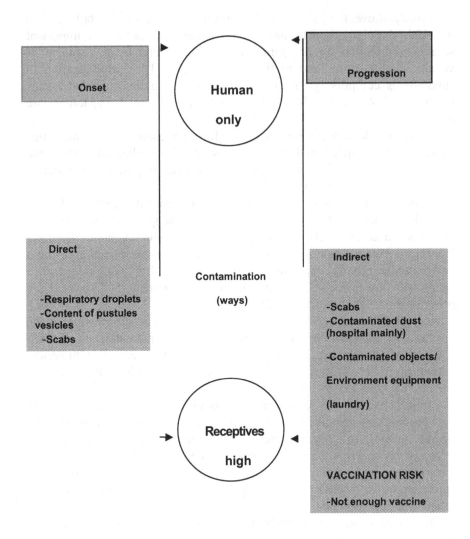

Figure 3. Epidemic risk factors in smallpox.

	Biosafety risk	Under the risk	Risk of contamination*
R	Hospital ↓	- Patients	- Clinical investigation - Procedures (therapeutic) - Sampling
I		- Personnel - Environment	- Death – manipulation - Waste- management
S	Sampling Transportation/ Manipulation ↓		- Laundry

K	Laboratory
	maximum
	containment
	(BL4)
		- Personnel
		- Environment
			- Procedures - investigation
			- Equipment - dedicated
			  Environment/negative
			  pressure

Figure 4. Smallpox: biosafety risk (extreme biosafety measures).

* Accidentally.

Air-conditioning plane systems activate the spreading of virus by respiratory route. Virus dispersion in the modern huge "crowded" plains is very "efficient" in contaminating hundreds of people at once. Potential sources (unknown contaminated persons) play a huge spreading risk.

Starting from a "first contaminated person" all the contacts incubating the smallpox become "secondary bioterrorists." Assuming a transmission rate of 20 cases by the "secondary bioterrorists" and a rate of 50 by the active, initial bioterrorist, a total of 1,000 cases would be prevalent before the earliest possible identification of the first wave of disease. Assuming that the first wave were misdiagnosed or diagnosed late the next wave would see 20,000 such cases, followed by 400,000 cases, 8 million cases, and so on [3].

Few physicians have enough experience, essential to establish a quick and accurate clinical diagnosis. But the high rapid detection and isolation of the first cases is crucial in limiting the risk of second-generation cases and in this context the professional training in urgent required today [3, 8, 12].

Preventing smallpox by vaccination is a long-debated decision. Well-known reverse reaction mentioned in Figure 3 is a major limiting risk factor in a mass vaccination campaign in the present situation. As WHO specialists recommended important stockpiles of specific globulin have to be prepared for the moment when the vaccination will be considered necessary [4, 15].

Biosafety biosecurity risk. Maximum security measures are recommended for special designated hospitals for isolation and quarantine for protection of personnel and environment. Negative air pressure, fully isolating equipment for personnel, and continuing disinfection measures are recommended for limiting the risk of contamination (Figure 4). Laundry and waste is sterilized and strictly surveyed for safety transportation before incineration [11].

Sample transportation and laboratories manipulating variola virus require maximum containment (BL4 biosafety) [3, 11].

Smallpox became a symbol of the victory of the humanity against infectious diseases. Risk assessment of smallpox estimated by many specialists after 2001 is an alarming scenario to prevent a global catastrophe, because epidemic extension of very aggressive diseases has no borders [1, 3, 14].

References

1. Alibek K. Biohazard. New York: Random House, 1999.
2. Alibek K. Smallpox: a disease and a weapon. Int J Infect Dis 2004; (Suppl 2): S3–S8.
3. Baxby D. Poxviruses. In: Collier L, Balows A, Jussmen M. Arnold (eds), Topley and Wilson's Microbiology and Microbial Infections, 9th edn. Vol. 1, London: Arnold, 1998, pp. 367–368.
4. Busch-Petersen E, Nagy E, Khouri PH. Smallpox – preparing for the emergency. Ellipse 2002; 18(3):57–68.
5. Cernescu C, Ruta S. Progrese in controlul si prevenirea virozelor cu potential bioterorist. Ed. Univ. Carol Davila, Bucuresti, 2004.
6. Ciufecu ES. Virusologie medicala. Ed. Medicala Nationala, Bucuresti, 2003.
7. Fauci SM. Foreword. In: Henderson AD, Inglesby VT, O'Toole T (eds), Bioterrorism: guidelines for medical and public health management. Chicago, IL: American Medical Association, 2002.
8. Ferguson NM, et al. Planning for smallpox: outbreak. Nature 2003; 425 (6959):681–685.
9. Henderson AD, Inglesby VT, Bartlett GJ, Ascher SM, Eitzen E, Jahrcing BP, Hauer J, Layton M, McDade J, Osterholm TM, O'Toole T, Parker G, Perl MT, Russell KP, Tonat K. Smallpox as a biological weapon. In: Henderson AD, Inglesby VT, O'Toole T (eds), Bioterrorism: guidelines for medical and public health management. Chicago, IL: American Medical Association, 1999.

10. Henderson AD. Smallpox biosecurity: preventing the unthinkable. London: Imperial College 2001.
11. Lalezari JR, Staag RJ, Kuppermann BD, et al. Intravenous cidofivir for peripheral cytomegalovirus retinitis in patients with AIDS a randomized, controlled trial. Ann Intern Med 1997; 126: 257–263.
12. Neff MJ. Variola (Smallpox) and Monkeypox viruses. In: Mandell LG, Bennet EJ, Dolin R (eds), Principle and practice of infectious diseases, 5th edn. Philadelphia: Churchill Livingstone, 2000.
13. Negut M. Preventing is better than postfactum intervention in bioerrorism. In: Gazso LG, Ponto CC (eds), Radiation inactivation of bioterrorism agents. Amsterdam: IOS Press, 2005, pp. 89–95.
14. Paun L. Variola (Variola Major). In: Amaltea (ed.), Boli infectioase, arme biologice, bioterorism. Bucuresti, 2003.
15. Ropp LS, Esposito JJ, Loparev NV, Palumbo JG. Poxvirus Infecting Humans. In: Murray PR, col. (eds), Manual of clinical microbiology, 7th edn. Washington, DC: ASM Press, 1999.
16. World Health Organization. The global eradication of smallpox. Final report of the Global commission for the certification of smallpox eradication. Geneva, Switzerland: WHO, 1980.

RENEWAL OF IMMUNOLOGICAL MEMORY TO SMALLPOX: USE OF NEW TOOLS YIELDS OLD RESULTS

Jonathan Boxman, Itay Wiser, and Nadav Orr
Center of Vaccine Development and Evaluation
Medical Corps, Israel Defense Forces

1. Abstract

The threat of smallpox, and with it smallpox vaccination, ended over 30 years ago. Since September 2001, a limited reintroduction of vaccination was carried out. The development of a skin reaction following vaccina vaccination ("take") remains the sole indicator of immunity acquisition.

Current vaccination policy states that immunity acquired from a one-time vaccination remains for less than 10 years and that individuals who fail to develop a "take" after revaccination must be rechallenged. However, historical records show smallpox resistance over 50 years after vaccination. Furthermore, recent studies have found that levels of vaccinia-specific B-cells and antibodies remain constant (after the decline of the initial reaction peak) over many decades while the T-cell levels steadily decline (half-life of 14 years) but are still identifiable for at least 50 years. A direct correlation has been observed between high anti-vaccinia antibody levels, immunity against vaccinia and variola, and lack of "take" during revaccination. These findings are strengthened by observations of immunity to vaccina illness in animals and humans lacking T-cell response (due to HIV syndrome or genetic defects), given high pre-exposure antibody levels.

This data indicates a central role for B-cells in maintaining immune protection from smallpox with a contributing role for T-cells as a memory component, and the problems inherent in determining the need for revaccination and evaluating new vaccines on the basis of the "take" indicator. Old and new findings have significant implications on evaluation of current herd immunity and prioritization in case of resumed vaccination.

Keywords:
Herd immunity, Immunological memory, Smallpox, Vaccinia, Vaccination.

M.S. Green et al. (eds.), Risk Assessment and Risk Communication Strategies in Bioterrorism Preparedness, 205–218.

2.   Background

The smallpox disease is distinguished in the long annals of medical history by a number of unique characteristics. This lethal disease that has claimed more victims than any other disease in human history is the first infection against which western medicine developed an effective cure, and is also the only human disease that has been completely eradicated, a goal that was achieved by 1979 due to an international effort led by the World Health Organization (WHO) [1, 2]. The disease was eradicated thanks to the use of a vaccinia inoculum, a genetic relative to the cowpox virus, whose utility in vaccinating against smallpox was first demonstrated at the end of the 18th century by Edward Janer.

Vaccination with the vaccinia inoculum is accompanied by a number of harmful side effects that posed a primary consideration in the decision to end routine smallpox vaccination. The events of September 11 and the anthrax letters led many governments to vaccinate medical personnel, as well as invest considerable resources in development of safer vaccines as a precautionary step against future bioterror attacks [3]. However, in spite of the immense resources invested in the revaccination campaign there is still no scientific consensus regarding the duration or mechanism of the immunity granted by the vaccina inoculum or the appropriate immunological parameters to investigate these questions [4].

Providing answers to these questions is important in several respects:

1. Estimating the time-related risk for smallpox infection in a population that had been previously vaccinated.
2. Determining parameters for the effectiveness of vaccination in a previously vaccinated population.
3. Determining parameters for the effectiveness of new vaccines.

The premise at the time of the smallpox eradication campaign was that vaccine-induced immunological memory to smallpox rapidly fades, with significant loss of protective immunity within 3–6 years [5, 6, 7, 8]. This concept was based on defining the appearance of a cutaneous response following the vaccination ("take") as the indication of a successful vaccination, and led to several US clinics recommending an annual vaccination to each patient, a tri-annual vaccination to all US citizens going abroad, and a compulsory vaccination of *Poxviridae* researchers every decade.

Several studies carried out prior to the smallpox eradication clearly indicate that the "take" symptoms were often observed in individuals receiving a booster vaccination shortly (several months) after the primary vaccination [4]. This would seem to indicate that the correlation between the "take" and the existence of systemic protective immunity is not high. How then can we determine the length of protective immunity granted by the vaccinia inoculum, the mechanism by which it is granted and the parameters suitable to measuring it?

Using Janer's original methods, namely infection of vaccinated individuals with the variola virus and analysis of the clinical results is not of course appropriate to this day and age but by carrying out an epidemiological analysis of prior smallpox outbreaks we can retrospectively reach conclusions regarding the duration of protective immunity. Furthermore, beyond the aspect of protective immunity to variola, the response and memory of the immune system to vaccinia poses an excellent model to study immunological memory thanks to several unique properties of the virus. First, vaccinia and variola do not chronically persist in their hosts – unlike other viruses such as EBC, Varicella, CMV, etc, [4] and do not, therefore, repeatedly stimulate the immune system. Furthermore, the eradication of the disease and the end of routine vaccinations means that any immunological parameters detected in individuals is the result of long-term immunological memory rather than random asyptomatic exposure.

3.   Historical Perspective

Janner originally claimed that the vaccinia inoculum provides full and indefinite protection versus smallpox [5]. His original report in 1798, concerning the development of protective immunity versus smallpox following infection with cowpox, included case reports demonstrating persistence of protective immunity for 25–38 years following exposure to cowpox. Janner recognized that critics might claim that this was caused by background exposure to variola (which was endemic at the time) and stated that "had these experiments been conducted in a large city, or in a populous neighborhood, some doubts might have been entertained; but here, where population is thin, and where such an event as a person's having had the smallpox is always faithfully recorded, no risk of inaccuracy in this particular can arise."

The duration of protective immunity remained a contention point and in his third study, published in 1800, Janner referred again to this point stating, "Some there are who suppose the security from the smallpox obtained through the cowpox will be of a temporary nature only. This supposition is refuted not only by analogy with respect to the habits of diseases of a similar nature, but by incontrovertible facts, which appear in great numbers against it . . . . But among the cases I refer to, one will be found of a person who had the cowpox fifty-three years before the effect of

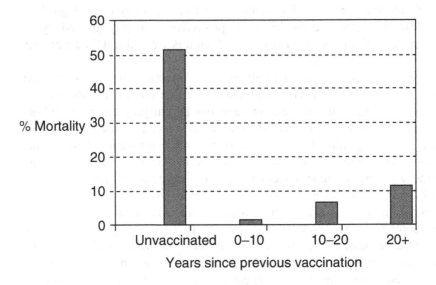

Figure 1. Mortality amongst European cases as presented by Mack et al. [11]. These figures refer to vaccinated individuals who were symptomatic to smallpox.

the smallpox was tried upon him. As he completely resisted it, the intervening period I conceive must necessarily satisfy any reasonable mind." Needless to say this example did not satisfy "every reasonable mind" in Janner's time and is certainly unsatisfactory today since the methodology of research and clinical record-keeping in use during the 18th century, combined with smallpox endemicity, render the quality of medical observations uncertain.

A study with higher standards describing a smallpox outbreak in Liverpool, England, was carried out in the early 19th century [9, 10]. Although there were common estimates regarding mortality from smallpox, no fatalities were identified among 206 cases of individuals who received a vaccination less than 20 years prior to the outbreak. Individuals who were vaccinated 20–30 years prior to the outbreak had a survival rate of 99% (330 out of 333), while the survival rate of individuals vaccinated 30–60 years prior to the outbreak was 94% (361 out of 384) (Figure 1). Obviously, since these studies were carried out when smallpox was still endemic in Europe, the study population may have been exposed to the virus prior to the outbreak. However, results from outbreaks in the 1950s and 1960s in European countries where the disease had been eradicated for over a generation showed remarkably similar results. These limited outbreaks ware caused by Third World immigrants and guest-workers who reintroduced variola to Europe (actually these outbreaks were a primary cause leading to the

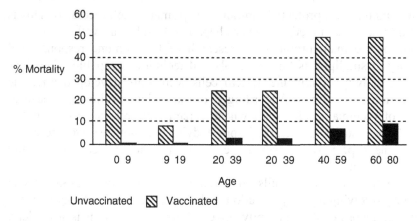

Figure 2. Morbidity and mortality data from smallpox outbreaks as presented by Hannah et al. [10]. The data refers to symptomatic individuals.

formation of the WHO smallpox eradication program and the willingness of the industrialized nations to fund the program), leading to a 55% mortality rate in the non-vaccinated European population [6, 9, 11]. However, individuals who were vaccinated over 20 years prior to the outbreak, and manifested clinical signs had a mortality rate of under 8% [9, 11] (Figure 2). It should be stressed that even this low mortality rateonly refers to vaccinated individuals who developed clinical symptoms of the disease (under 4% of contacts) [11]. Therefore, the survival rate of individuals who were exposed to the disease more than 20 years after their previous vaccination was over 99%. The data from these historical studies was recently incorporated in a mathematical model predicting long-term protective immunity to smallpox [9]. The creators of the model claim that these results indicate that although protection from infection does decline in time, protection from severe illness resulting in death remains indefinitely – as Janner originally claimed (Figure 1).

3.1.   MECHANISMS OF PROTECTIVE IMMUNITY FORMATION AND MAINTENANCE TO SMALLPOX

The relative importance of the humoral and cellular components of the immune system in providing protection from smallpox and mechanism by which this immunity is maintained remains a subject of fierce contention with significant implications for the length of protective immunity granted by vaccination. Smallpox's long period of presymptomatic incubation (two weeks) provides a long stretch of time for T and B memory cells to expand and activate the mechanisms required to contain the infection, reinforcing the assumption that protective immunity is primarily cell mediated. This is true for other viral infections such as hepatitis A and B, as well.

One of the main problems in research of the immune response and memory to smallpox is that the tools and techniques capable of evaluating the activity of immune system cells were only developed after the eradication of smallpox. Accordingly, our knowledge relies on measurements of vaccinia specific cells whose veracity and relevance is doubtful. Nonetheless, much can be learned from studying the immune system response to vaccinia, especially by analyzing cases of immunodefecient patients and laboratory animals.

The importance of T-cells in generation of immune response and memory following primary infection with variola remains indisputable, but their role in protective immunity upkeep versus reinfection is less clear. Mouse and ape models showed that T-cells were not required for protection from vaccinia if antibodies to the virus were already present [12, 13]. An in-depth analysis of the relative contribution of the various components of the immune system to protective immunity upkeep has only recently become feasible thanks to the application of techniques permitting direct visualization and analysis of antigen specific T- and B-cells [13, 14, 15, 16, 17, 18].

4.   T-cell-Mediated Antiviral Memory

T-cells are regarded as the primary mediators of long-term immunological memory, but while their vital importance in the generation of immune response and memory following primary infection is indisputable [18], their role in protective immunity upkeep has been rendered uncertain by a number of recent studies. A study carried out in US volunteers who were previously vaccinated 1–14 times revealed that the number of vaccinia antigen-specific T-cells declines with a half-life of 8–15 years – regardless of the number of booster vaccinations. The rate of decline of CD4+ cells summed to be lower than that of CD8+ cells but remarkably vaccinia-specific T-cells of both types could still be detected in some individuals 75 years postvaccination.

Similar results were acquired in a study following up vaccinia-specific T-cell levels 50 years postvaccination. The T-cell half-life estimated from the results was 14 years [14]. These results also match measurements indicating a higher level of precursors to vaccinia-specific CD4+ memory cells than CD8+ memory cells 35 years postvaccination, and to another study where researchers encountered considerable difficulties in isolating CD8+ but not CD4+ T-cells 20 years postvaccination [19].

It is noteworthy that in contrast to these results, a murine model of lymphocytic choriomeningitis virus (LCMV) infection showed a far longer maintenance of CD8+ T-cells than CD4+ T-cells. It is unclear whether this variance is the result of differences in the host, the virus, or the study methods [20]. However, considering that *Poxviridae* are commonly transported from the lungs to the rest of the body by major histocompatibility complex type II (MHCII) displaying phagocytic cells and that respiratory epithelial cells often display MHCII, a central role for MHCII recognizing CD4+ T-cells in maintaining the long-term protective immunity to smallpox seems plausible [21].

5.   B-cell-Mediated Antiviral Memory

Antibodies are the immune system's first line of defense against infections. Indeed, antibody levels are the most widely used parameter of estimating the formation of protective immunity in most human vaccines [22]. Plentiful evidence exists for the involvement of long-lived plasma cells in the upkeep of antibody levels and of memory cells in the formation of the secondary response upon reexposure. Memory B-cells may also play a role in refreshing the long-lived plasma cell repertoire even in the absence of exposure to antigen stimulation [22].

What is the importance of vaccinia-specific antibody level in providing protective immunity from smallpox? Ape models (Rhesus macaque) demonstrated that the outcome of primary infection of both healthy and simian immunodeficiency virus (SIV) was in correlation to CD4+ T-cell levels. In contrast, no correlation between CD4+ T-cell levels was observed in secondary infection, rather, a powerful correlation was observed to with the pre-infection level of vaccinia-specific antibodies [13]. Likewise, a murine model of intranasal vaccinia infection showed T-cells to be vital in the generation of an initial immune response following primary infection but the subsequent neutralization of CD4+/CD8+ T-cells had no effect on the outcome of secondary infection – provided a high level of anti-vaccina antibodies was still present in the bloodstream [12].

Human studies performed in the 1950s showed that of individuals inoculated with vaccinia who then showed clinical signs of smallpox, the mortality rate of low responders (as measured by antibody levels) was 33% versus only 5.6% of high responders [4]. The correlation between antibody levels and resistance to smallpox was demonstrated again in two independent studies published in the early 1970s indicating that individuals with prevaccination antibody levels of >1:20 were better protected from smallpox infection [5, 23].

The dynamics of antigen-specific memory B-cells in the absence of reexposure to the antigen is not clearly understood. Smallpox vaccine offers a unique opportunity to explore this issue due to the eradication of the disease and the prolonged period since the last vaccinations. This opportunity has been utilized by a number of research groups [14, 17] who discovered that antibody and memory B-cell levels tend to stabilize following the decline of the initial peak and remain constant indefinitely (over 75 years).

This dynamic is quite different from that of the T-cells, whose level declines at a constant rate with a half-life of 14 years [17]. Not only do the antibody levels to vaccinia remain constant and high in the vaccinee sera, the memory B-cells maintain a capability for rapid production of antibodies (20-fold increase) following reexposure to the vaccinia antigen [14]. Although booster vaccinations have led to a rapid and powerful antibody response, antibody levels maintained following the decline of the initial peak were only slightly improved by a second vaccination, with no improvements whatsoever following additional booster vaccinations. This indicates that while booster vaccinations may raise antibody levels achieved from a suboptimal response, there is a physiological limitation to the amount of antibodies an individual may maintain against any given antigen.

The mechanism behind the long-term maintenance of antibody production may be the result of activation/differentiation of memory B-cells, the survival of long-lived plasma cells, or a combination of all of these factors [14]. Long-term maintenance of vaccinia-specific B-cells and antibodies on near-constant levels is consistent with the immunological memory characteristics observed from epidemiological historical background of the disease – a consistency in dictating a major role for the humoral portion of the immune system in maintaining protective immunity from reinfection by *Poxviridae* viruses (Figure 3).

Data indicating the importance of pre-exposure antibody levels were also found in an Israel Defense Forces (IDF) Medical Corps study carried out in the context of a revaccination campaign versus smallpox [21]. An inverse correlation was found between the prevaccination vaccinia specific antibody levels and seroconversion (fourfold rise in antibody levels) cutaneous reaction ("take") following the vaccination (Figure 4). It can be deduced that individuals with high initial antibody levels suppressed the vaccinia infection at an early stage prior to the development of clinical symptoms and without the involvement of memory cells. Similar results were achieved in a study carried out in the National Institute of Allergy and Infectious Diseases in St. Louis, USA [16].

6.   Discussion

The academic and emotional controversy regarding the danger and need to vaccinate versus smallpox has resulted in a wide reappraisal of fundamental issues in immunological memory development and upkeep. When Janner developed the smallpox vaccine, he had neither the knowledge base nor the molecular tools to define the mechanisms by which his vaccine induced immunological memory. Furthermore, the methodology of clinical record-keeping was not sufficiently prevalent, reliable, or uniform to evaluate the effectiveness of the vaccine, especially given the endemicity of the disease. Lacking the tools to directly measure the vaccina components of the immune system, or the records to correlate them with protective immunity, the cutaneous response ("take") was selected as the parameter for postvaccination development of protective immunity. Unable to evaluate the long-term effectiveness of the vaccine, and facing an epidemic claiming many lives each year, the world's medical authorities chose to recommend frequent booster vaccination, a policy that remained unchanged until the eradication of the disease in 1979. The events of September 11 reopened the public discourse and led to a large number of studies reanalyzing epidemiological data from the heyday of the smallpox eradication campaign and utilizing the new molecular tools to evaluate the humoral and cellular parameters associated with protective immunity to smallpox.

The juxtaposition of these conditions now permits us, without the constant pressure an endemic plague asserted on earlier decision maker, to reevaluate smallpox vaccination policy in light of the new-old data emerging from these studies:

1.   Epidemiological analysis of the imported smallpox outbreaks of the 1950s in Europe and Liverpool, England 1902, indicate that a single vaccination provides a protective immunity of over 93% for 20+ years (Figure 3) [9, 10, 11].
2.   The number of vaccinia-specific memory B-cells remains stable over several years in individuals who were vaccinated more than 50 years ago – and they in turn maintained a steady level of vaccinia-specific antibodies [13, 14, 17] (Figure 3).
3.   There is a significant correlation between the outcome of vaccinia/variola infection and antibody levels [23, 24].

4. The number of vaccinia-specific T-cells declines after initial exposure (half-life of 14 years) but can still be recognized after several decades [14, 15, 17, 19].
5. No direct correlation between vaccinia-specific T- and B-cell levels (and antibody levels) [13].
6. Protective immunity to vaccinia is provided by high levels of specific antibodies even with no T-cell activity [12, 13, 18].

Although many of these findings relate to vaccinia rather than variola, the weight of evidence indicates that current smallpox vaccinations provide protection from mortality to the overwhelming majority of the population for over 50 years. This protection is primarily mediated by memory B-cells and long-lived plasma cells and to some extent by T-cells, as well. What that are the operative conclusions that may be drawn from these assumptions?

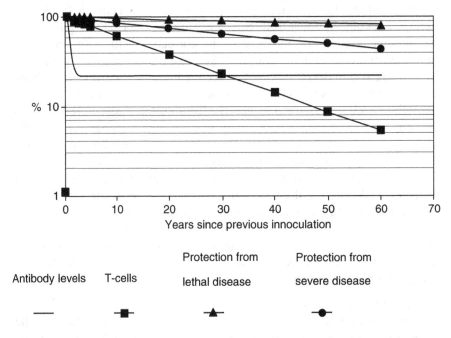

Figure 3. Diminishment of immune memory in time. Data has been taken from two independent studies [14, 17] with similar results. All antibodies specific to vaccinia stabilized after the decline of the initial peak on levels that did not significantly change throughout life. T-cell levels, however, decline at a half-life of 14 [14] or 8–15 years [17]. The rate of immune protection decline has been calculated by Eichner [9] based on reports from Liverpool outbreak in 1902 [10] in the European outbreaks of 1950–1971 [11].

6.1.   VACCINATION: INDIVIDUAL AND PUBLIC HEALTH CONSIDERATIONS

The difficulties in establishing a direct linkage between immune parameters to vaccinia and mortality from variola inhibit the use of antibody levels/cellular activity to determine the protective immunity of an individual. Certainly, statistical analysis indicating low mortality in previously vaccinated individuals shall not prevent individuals from seeking booster vaccinations in case of a smallpox alert. However, high protective immunity within a previously vaccinated population subgroup may determine vaccination priorities during a smallpox outbreak or alert and in providing booster vaccinations to individuals who do not develop a "take." In this context revaccinating previously vaccinated individuals in order to reduce side effects may be redundant since protective immunity among this population is already high.

Furthermore, the implications of prolonged protective immunity on the speed of smallpox expansion in the general population and the public health interventions necessary to contain it should be considered. One of the primary parameters for assessing the risk of spread of smallpox in the general population is R_0, the average number of secondary cases infected by a primary case. Obviously the value of R_0 is directly correlated with the herd immunity of the exposed population. While the existing models [6, 7, 8, 25] dispute both the R_0 in historical outbreaks and the expected R_0 from a bioterror attack on western targets all rely on the Centers for Disease Control and Prevention (CDC) stance regarding the rapid decline of vaccine efficacy, and therefore estimate vaccine protective immunity at 18% in the UK and 20% in the United States. If protective immunity actually persists for 30+ years as epidemiological investigations of historical outbreaks indicate (Chart 3), a far larger proportion of the population may be affected with smallpox spread being correspondingly slower.

6.2.   PARAMETER FOR SUCCESS OF VACCINATION

The cutaneous reaction ("take") to the vaccinia compound, serves as the sole accepted parameter for the success of smallpox vaccination. The "take" is apparently a combination of the immune response to vaccinia and damage caused from the spread of the virus and cell destruction around the site of inoculation. Over the past years several researchers have demonstrated that lack of "take" upon revaccination is not an indication for failed vaccination but rather of preexisting protective immunity that eliminates the vaccinia virus before it can multiply. Therefore, the cost benefit of revaccinating individuals who do not develop a "take" (40% of revaccinated individuals) should be reconsidered.

6.3.   EVALUATING VACCINES

Among the primary causes of ending standard vaccinations to smallpox was the frequency of negative side effects. These side effects are strongly associated with the cutaneous "take" used as a parameter of the vaccine's success. Accordingly, relying on the "take" to asses new vaccines that are supposed to reduce side effects by attenuating the virus is problematic. Seroconversion or T/B-cell proliferation may prove to be a better and more reliable parameter of judging the effectiveness of new vaccines.

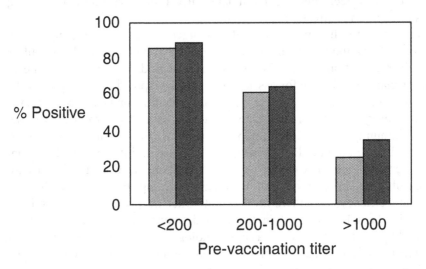

Figure 4. Effect of prevaccination titer on portion of vaccinees who undergo seroconversion or develop "take." (From Orr et al. [24].)

References

1. CDC. 25th anniversary of the last case of naturally acquired smallpox. MMWR 2002; 51:952.
2. Eyler JM. Smallpox in history: the birth death and impact of a dread disease. J lab Clin Med 142(4):216–220.
3. Wright ME, Fauci AS. Smallpox immunization in the 21st century, the old and the new. JAMA Jun 25, 2003; 289(24):3306–3308.

4. Slifka MK. Immunological memory to viral infection. Curr Opin Immunol 2004 Aug; 16(4):443–450.
5. Bray M. New data in a 200-year investigation. Clin Infect Dis 2004 Jan 1; 38(1):90–91. Epub Dec 8, 2003. No abstract available.
6. Gani R, Leach S. Transmission potential of smallpox in contemporary populations. Nature 2001; 414:748–751.
7. Meltzer MI, Damon I, LeDuc JW, Millar JD. Modeling potential responses to smallpox as a bioterrorist weapon. Emerg Infect Dis 2001; 7:959–969.
8. O'Toole T, Mair M, Inglesby TV. Shining light on "Dark Winter". Clin Infect Dis 2002; 34:972–983.
9. Eichner M. Analysis of historical data suggests long-lasting protective effects of smallpox vaccination. Am J Epidemiol 2003; 158:717–723.
10. Hanna W, Baxby D. Studies in smallpox and vaccination. 1913. Rev Med Virol 2002; 12(4):201–209.
11. Mack TM. Smallpox in Europe, 1950–1971. J Infect Dis 1972; 125:161–169.
12. Belyakov IM, Earl P, Dzutsev A, Kuznetsov VA, Lemon M, Wyatt LS, Snyder JT, Ahlers JD, Franchini G, Moss B et al. Shared modes of protection against poxvirus infection by attenuated and conventional smallpox vaccine viruses. Proc Natl Acad Sci USA 2003; 100:9458–9463.
13. Edghill-Smith Y, Venzon D, Karpova T, McNally J, Nacsa J, Tsai WP, Tryniszewska E, Moniuszko M, Manischewitz J, King LR et al. Modeling a safer smallpox vaccination regimen, for human immunodeficiency virus type 1-infected patients, in immunocompromised macaques. J Infect Dis 2003; 188:1181–1191.
14. Crotty S, Felgner P, Davies H, Glidewell J, Villarreal L, Ahmed R. Cutting Edge: long-term B cell memory in humans after smallpox vaccination. J Immunol 2003; 171:4969–4973.
15. Demkowicz WEJ, Littaua RA, Wang J, Ennis FA. Human cytotoxic T-cell memory: long-lived responses to vaccinia virus. J Virol 1996; 70:2627–2631.
16. Frey SE, Newman FK, Yan L, Belshe RB, Response to smallpox vaccine in persons immunized in the distant past. JAMA 2003; 289:3295–3299.
17. Hammarlund E, Lewis MW, Hansen SG, Strelow LI, Nelson JA, Sexton GJ, Hanifin JM, Slifka MK. Duration of antiviral immunity after smallpox vaccination. Nature Medicine 2003; 9(9):1131–1137.
18. Xu R, Johnson AJ, Liggitt D, Bevan MJ. Cellular and humoral immunity against vaccinia virus infection of mice. Immunol 2004 May 15; 172(10): 6265–6271.
19. Erickson AL, Walker CM. Class I major histocompatibility complex-restricted cytotoxic T cell responses to vaccinia virus in humans. J Gen Virol 1993; 74:751–754.
20. Homann D, Teyton L, Oldstone MB. Differential regulation of antiviral T-cell immunity results in stable CD8+ but declining CD4+ T-cell memory. Nat Med 2001; 7:913–919.

21. Hegde NR, Johnson DC. Human cytomegalovirus US2 causes similar effects on both major histocompatibility complex class I and II proteins in epithelial and glial cells. J Virol 2003; 77:9287–9294.

22. Crotty S, Ahmed R. Immunological memory in humans. Semin Immunol 2004 Jun; 16(3):197–203. Review.

23. Mack TM, Noble J Jr, Thomas DB. A prospective study of serum antibody and protection against smallpox. Am J Trop Med Hyg 1972; 21:214–218.

24. Orr N, Forman M, Marcus H, Lustig S, Paran N, Grotto I, Klement E,Yehezkelli Y, Robin G, Reuveny S, Shafferman A, Cohen D. Vaccinia Study Group, Medical Corps, Israel Defense Force; Vaccinia Study Group, Israel Institute for Biological Research. Clinical and immune responses after revaccination of Israeli adults with the Lister strain of vaccinia virus. J Infect Dis 2004 Oct 1; 190(7):1295–1302. Epub Aug 30, 2004.

25. Kaplan EH, Craft DL, Wein LM. Emergency response to a smallpox attack: the case for mass vaccination. Proc Natl Acad Sci USA 2002; 99:10935–10940.

PREPARING FOR A SMALLPOX BIOTERRORIST ATTACK: PULSE VACCINATION AS AN OPTIMAL STRATEGY

Zvia Agur[1], Karen Marron[1], Hanita Shai[1],
and Yehuda L. Danon[2]
[1]*Institute for Medical BioMathematics (IMBM)*
10 Hate'ena St.; P.O.B. 282, 60991
Bene Ataroth, Israel
[2]*Kipper Institute of Immunology*
Schneider Children Medical Center; FMRC
Petach-Tikva, 49202; Israel

1.   Introduction

Events of recent years have significantly increased our awareness of the potential threat of a bioterrorist attack, and the smallpox variola virus has been identified as an "eligible candidate" for a biological warfare agent. Epidemiological mathematical modeling has long been recognized as a crucial tool for assessing the repercussions of such a viral outbreak, as well as for comparing possible response strategies. Several studies have applied mathematical models with the hope of identifying an optimal vaccination strategy in case of an attack [1–4]. However, these particular studies do not produce clear-cut recommendations, upon which authorities can rely when formulating policies. In fact, conclusions of certain studies contradict those of others.

This inconsistency may stem from simulation results' extreme sensitivity to the value assumed for the disease's basic reproduction rate (R_0) [5], i.e., the number of secondary infections that an infectious individual is expected to produce if introduced into an entirely susceptible population. Because smallpox was eradicated in 1979, there is a lack of current epidemiological data on the disease, and R_0 must be estimated. However, as this value is dependent both on biological factors and on population dynamics, it is extremely difficult to assess prior to an actual epidemic. Each of the above-mentioned studies assumes a different value for R_0, which may account for their contradictory results: a response strategy found

M.S. Green et al. (eds.), Risk Assessment and Risk Communication Strategies in Bioterrorism
Preparedness, 219-229.
© 2007 *Springer.*

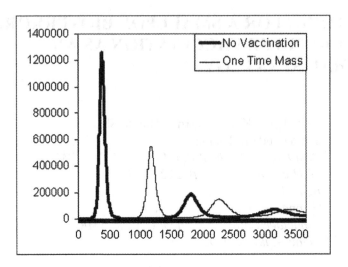

Figure 1. Simulation results of the adapted the susceptible, exposed, infectious, recovered (SEIR) model: Number of infected individuals over time when disease is introduced into the Israeli population by one infective carrier.
Thick line: Natural disease dynamics (no vaccination strategy is implemented).
Thin line: Disease dynamics after implementation of *one-time mass vaccination* strategy (population is vaccinated at maximum capacity for 3 days following the attack).

to be effective in the case of a low disease transmission rate may fall short when faced with a higher transmission rate.

Furthermore, there is a fundamental limitation that compromises the practical value of theoretical smallpox studies to date: they examine response strategies that address only an initial epidemic, without considering long-term effects of the introduction of the disease into a contemporary population. Theory indicates that smallpox, like many other contagious diseases, is characterized by decaying oscillatory dynamics, i.e., periodic epidemics of decreasing magnitude [6]. Thus, while a given vaccination strategy may succeed in curbing an outbreak immediately following the release of the virus it may not be able to prevent additional epidemics several years down the line (Figure 1). Clearly, an efficient follow-up strategy is no less important than initial crisis aversion. Nevertheless, most smallpox studies either fail to mention such a strategy, or simply assume that the entire population will continue to be vaccinated in the years following the outbreak. This type of continuous vaccination policy would be far from optimal, as vaccinia, the smallpox vaccine, is known to cause serious, and even fatal, side effects. Additionally, the vaccine carries quite a few contraindications: for example, it is not recommended to administer it to young children [6]. Due to these significant constraints, it becomes evident that a general idea for a long-term vaccination strategy is insufficient; this strategy must be rigorously defined. Theory implies that efficient control of phenomena, such as smallpox transmission, which display clear periodicity, should involve a *periodic* strategy with a period different from that of the phenomenon being counteracted [7, 8].

Based on these guidelines, we examine a vaccination strategy that has not yet been considered in the context of response to a smallpox bioterrorist attack: *pulse vaccination*, i.e., periodic vaccination of certain percentages of the susceptible population following attack. The *pulse* strategy has previously been proposed as an efficient method for measles eradication [9, 10]. In addition to its theoretically proven efficacy, this strategy also enables flexibility: the number of people vaccinated and the duration of time between vaccination campaigns (inter-vaccination interval) can be varied according to arising circumstances. This flexibility is crucial when dealing with a situation as sensitive as a smallpox bioterrorist attack, with so many unknown and unpredictable factors, e.g., the disease's actual basic reproduction rate, the population's response to an outbreak and willingness to comply with vaccination campaigns, available vaccine stockpile, vaccine efficacy, etc.

In this study, we compare the *pulse vaccination* strategy to two known smallpox response strategies: (i) *preliminary vaccination*, i.e., vaccination of a certain percentage of the population prior to the attack; (ii) *one-time mass vaccination*, in which most of the population is vaccinated immediately following the attack. Additional vaccination strategies that have been considered for smallpox protection are *trace* and *ring vaccination*, in which vaccination is limited to close contacts of infected individuals. Though these approaches are potentially effective in large countries [11], they are not considered feasible in small countries with high population density such as Israel, and therefore we did not include them in our study.

To compare the performance of the different vaccination strategies under a wide range of conditions, we adapted the susceptible, exposed, infectious, recovered (SEIR) epidemiological model [6] to describe the effects of a smallpox bioterrorist attack on the Israeli population over a period of 10 years. We simulate and compare the different vaccination strategies under the constraints of low compliance, insufficient vaccine stockpile, contraindications, side effects, cost of vaccination, etc. In order to obtain robust conclusions, we evaluate the performance of each studied vaccination strategy over a wide range of potential basic reproduction rate (R_0) values $(1.5 \leq R_0 \leq 30)$.

It is important to note that though these simulations were carried out with smallpox in mind, the results are applicable to almost any infectious disease.

2.   Mathematical Modeling

We adapted a classic SEIR model for the transmission of an infectious disease in a spatially heterogeneous population [6]. We assume that the smallpox virus is introduced into the Israeli population by one infective carrier. The model takes into account three stages of infection [12], assuming that each stage has a constant duration (d_1, d_2, and d_3 in Table 1 respectively): (1) infected, noninfective, and vaccine sensitive; (2) infected, noninfective, vaccine-insensitive; (3) infected and infective. We define the basic transmission rate as: $\beta = \dfrac{R_0}{Nd_3}$, where N is the initial population size. A certain fraction of infective cases die of the disease, and the remaining fraction eventually recovers, becoming immune to reinfection. The model does not consider loss of immunity following vaccination or recovery from the disease [13].

TABLE 1. Model parameters

Parameter	Value	Unit	Reference
Initial susceptible population	6,439,200	Individuals	
Initial infective population	1	Individual	
Birth rate	$9e^{-4}$		
Death rate	$9e^{-4}$		
First stage disease duration (d_1)	4	Days	[12]
Second stage disease duration (d_2)	13	Days	[12]
Third stage disease duration (d_3)	21	Days	[12]
Disease fatality rate	0.3		[12]
Vaccine fatality rate	10^{-6}		[12]
Rate of non-fatal vaccination side effects	0.001		[12]
Maximum daily vaccination capacity	$1.8e^{6}$	Individuals	
Duration of pulse vaccination campaign	3	Days	

We examine three vaccination policies as follows: (i) *Preliminary vaccination*: Different percentages of the population are vaccinated prior to attack, from 0% to 100% in increments of 5%; (ii) *One-time mass vaccination*: We define a "maximum vaccination capacity," i.e., the maximum number of people that can be vaccinated per day (Table 1). The percentage of capacity utilized (PCU) is varied between 0% and 100% in increments of 5%, and the duration of the vaccination campaign is varied between 1 and 15 days in increments of 1 day; (iii) *Pulse vaccination*: PCU is varied from 0% to 100% in increments of 5%, and the interval between cycles is varied from 50 to 2000 days in increments of 50 days. Due to computational considerations, the duration of periodic vaccination campaigns is set as constant (3 days).

When applying *one-time mass vaccination* or *pulse vaccination* strategies, priority is given to individuals who have been exposed to the disease but can still be effectively vaccinated.

3.   Strategy Assessment: The "Cost" of An Outbreak

Theoretically, continuous vaccination of the entire population would be a foolproof means of preventing disease outbreak. However, as previously mentioned, this would not be the optimal strategy, due to the constraints imposed by the vaccinia vaccine [12]. In addition, it would probably not be reasonable to expect full compliance, especially over a long period of time after the initial outbreak. Therefore, an optimal strategy should not only prevent disease outbreak, but should allow as few individuals as possible to be vaccinated.

Vaccinating fewer individuals will not only prevent side effects, but will be less disruptive to routine. Thus, in order to assess the efficacy of a particular strategy, we determine a "cost," which takes into account the following factors: (i) number of deaths by infection (D_{inf}); (ii) number of infections (I); (iii) number of people vaccinated (N_{vac}); (iv) number of deaths resulting from vaccination (D_{vac}); (v) non-fatal side effects of vaccination (E); and (vi) a "stress factor": number of post-attack vaccinations performed per day (S).

Each factor is attributed a "weight," and the cost C is calculated as follows: $C = (WD_{inf} + \dfrac{W}{2}I + N_{vac} + \dfrac{W}{10}E + 2WD_{vac})(1 + Se^{-7})$.

Where W is an "anchor weight," which represents the ratio between the weight of death by infection and the number of vaccinees. This value can be interpreted as the number of individuals a country is willing to vaccinate in order to save one life. Clearly, the resulting cost is closely dependent on the value of these weights. Therefore, to obtain robust results, we run simulations over a wide range of "anchor weights" (range: 1–10,000).

Model parameters are presented in Table 1, where demographic parameters apply to the Israeli population. Additional parameter values, such as disease phase duration, etc. are taken from classic references. Clearly, disease and vaccine fatality rates are extremely influential when determining the trade-off between the number of vaccinees and the number of deaths by disease. The model's possible sensitivity to these parameters is accounted for by varying the "anchor weight" applied when computing the cost (see above). As previously mentioned, a crucial parameter for assessing the effects of an outbreak is R_0. However, this parameter is also extremely difficult to estimate, as it is dependent on dynamic factors, such as socioeconomic conditions [6, 12]. The basic transmission rate of smallpox has been estimated between 3 and 10 [14, 15], and values implemented in studies vary between 1.5 and 15 [2, 3]. Instead of assuming a single value for R_0, we run simulations over a wide range of values, which vary between 1.5 and 30.

3.1.   RESULTS

As previously described, we simulated and compared various applications of *preliminary, one-time mass vaccination,* and *pulse vaccination* strategies. Each simulated strategy design produced a final cost, a low cost signifying an efficient strategy, and a relatively high cost signifying an inefficient strategy. Figure 2 presents the distribution of costs attained by each strategy simulated, for several values of R_0. Different costs for the same strategy are achieved by varying strategy design (e.g., a *preliminary vaccination* strategy in which 75% of the population is vaccinated may produce a lower cost than a *preliminary* strategy in which only 20% of the population is vaccinated). Figure 2 indicates that for $R_0 \geq 1.5$, all three vaccination strategies tested can potentially be efficient: if properly designed, they can reduce "cost" to zero. However, for $R_0 > 1.5$, *pulse vaccination* is the only strategy that succeeds in minimizing cost. This result holds true even for $R_0 > 10$, i.e., beyond the range of values that have been estimated. The same qualitative results are obtained even when the "anchor weight" is varied, provided that the weight chosen indicates vaccination to be preferable over non-vaccination (Figure 3).

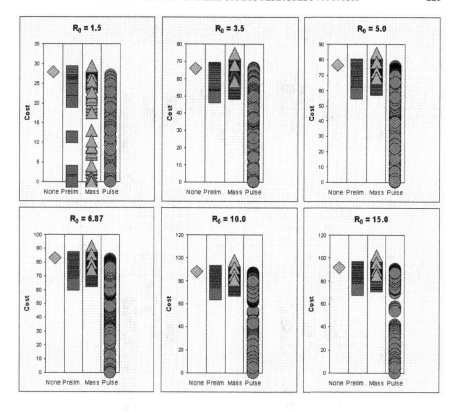

Figure 2. Costs produced by each simulated vaccination strategy for several values of R_0. Strategies tested: *preliminary vaccination* (squares), *one-time mass vaccination* (triangles), and *pulse vaccination* (circles). Different costs for the same strategy are obtained by varying strategy design.

3.2.   PULSE VACCINATION: FINDING THE OPTIMAL DESIGN

Though *pulse vaccination* can potentially be an effective strategy, inappropriate strategy design is likely to produce high costs (Figure 2). Therefore it is crucial to identify the optimal strategy design, in terms of PCU and the interval between "pulses." Figure 4 presents graphs of cost as a function of PCU and interval between pulses for several values of R_0.

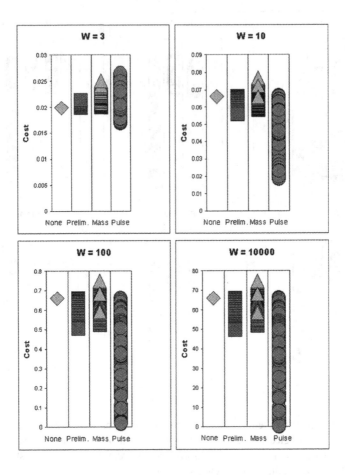

Figure 3. Costs produced by each simulated vaccination strategy for several values of the anchor weight (W = 3; 10; 100; R_0 is 3.5). As in Figure 2, strategies tested are *preliminary vaccination* (squares), *one-time mass vaccination* (triangles), and *pulse vaccination* (circles). Note that for W = 3, *pulse vaccination* is not more efficient than other strategies, but at the same time non-vaccination is as efficient as vaccination. For larger W values, *pulse vaccination* is more efficient.

As is evident from these graphs, for each R_0 value there is a "zone" (shaded areas) in which costs are low, and outside of which costs rise suddenly. This zone is defined by a diagonal contour, which means that there is a critical ratio of PCU to interval between pulses above which the *pulse* strategy will effectively reduce costs, and below which the strategy is inefficient. This critical ratio increases in direct relation to R_0 (Figure 5).

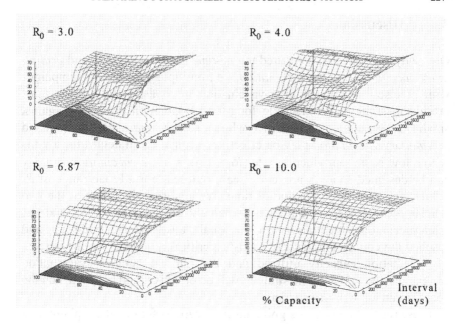

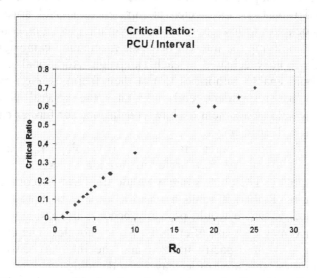

Figure 4. Pulse vaccination: Cost as a function of percent vaccination capacity utilized and interval (in days) between pulses, for several R_0 values. There is a critical ratio (diagonal contour) between the two, above which the strategy will be effective (shaded area) and below which costs rise suddenly.

Figure 5. There is a critical ratio of percent vaccination capacity utilized to interval between pulses that must be exceeded in order for a *pulse* strategy to be effective. *In graph*: Critical ratio as a function of R_0.

4.   Discussion

Our study suggests that compared to *one-time mass vaccination* and *preliminary vaccination*, *pulse vaccination*, i.e., multiple vaccination campaigns with precisely calculated inter-vaccination intervals, is by far the most promising strategy for ensuring long-term population protection against smallpox. Simulations show that while *one-time mass vaccination* and *preliminary vaccination* may be effective vaccination strategies for a virus with a low basic reproduction rate ($R_0 \leq 1.5$), a *pulse vaccination* strategy can be designed so as to prevent disease outbreak for a broad range of R_0 values, and over a long period of time. We analyzed the effect of the two crucial *pulse* strategy parameters – namely the coverage level and the inter-vaccination intervals – on the final "cost" of the outbreak, and reached the conclusion that there exists a critical ratio between the percent of vaccination capacity utilized and the interval between vaccination campaigns above which the strategy will be effective, and below which the "cost" of attack will rise suddenly.

These results may carry significant implications for countries planning a response to a smallpox bioterrorist attack, or to an outbreak of any disease for which a vaccine exists, but about which little else is known. They indicate that given the realistic range of the disease's basic reproduction rate and the estimated compliance level, authorities can design a detailed, optimal vaccination plan for years to come. This plan would be extremely flexible and robust: if unexpected circumstances should arise, e.g., insufficient stockpiles or low compliance, maximum protection could still be ensured by modifying the interval between vaccination campaigns, or the number of people vaccinated at each campaign. Additionally, the pulse strategy would enable authorities to test their facilities, e.g., by initially vaccinating first responders, and only later the general public. This preparation would allow them to draw conclusions for further campaigns, increasing overall efficiency.

Clearly, for both bureaucratic and psychological reasons, the government of a country may prefer to provide a mass or preliminary vaccination policy. The pulse strategy would not have to replace either of these strategies. Rather, it could be used as a backup strategy, and as a long-term policy, which would probably become increasingly necessary, as compliance may decrease after initial panic subsides. The critical ratio between the percent capacity utilized and the interval between pulses offers authorities quite a bit of leeway when deciding upon the timing and the magnitude of these campaigns.

Acknowledgments

This work was supported in part by the Chai Foundation, and in part by the Israeli Defense Forces.

References

1. Meltzer MI, Damon I, LeDuc JW, Millar JD. Modeling potential responses to smallpox as a bioterrorist weapon. Emerg Infect Dis 2001; 7:959–969.
2. Kaplan EH, Craft DL, Wein LM. Emergency response to a smallpox attack: the case for mass vaccination. Proc Natl Acad Sci USA 2002; 99:10935–10940.
3. Bozette SA, Boer R, Bhatnagar V, Brower JL, Keeler E, Morton SC, et al. A model for a smallpox-vaccination policy. N Engl J Med 2002; 348:416–425.
4. Halloran ME, Longini IM, Nizham A, Yang Y. Containing bioterrorist smallpox. Science 2002; 298:1428–1432.
5. Ferguson NM, Keeling MJ, Edmunds WJ, Gani R, Grenfell BT, Anderson RM et al. Nature. Planning for smallpox outbreaks 2003; 425:681–685.
6. Anderson RM, May RM. Infectious diseases of humans: dynamics and control. Oxford: Oxford University Press, 1991.
7. Agur, Z. Randomness, synchrony and population persistence. J Theor Biol 1985; 112:677–693.
8. Agur, Z. Resonance and anti-resonance in the design of chemotherapeutic protocols. J Theor Med 1998; 1:237–245.
9. Agur Z, Cojocaru L, Mazor G, Anderson RM, Danon YL. Pulse mass measles vaccination across age cohorts. Proc Natl Acad Sci USA 1993; 90:11698–11702.
10. Shulgin B, Stone L, Agur Z. Pulse vaccination strategy in the SIR epidemic model. Bull Math Biol 1998; 60(6):1123–1148.
11. Fraser C, Riley S, Anderson RM, Ferguson N. Factors that make an infectious disease outbreak controllable. PNAS 2004; 101:6146–6151.
12. Fenner F, Henderson DA, Arita I, Jezek Z, Ladnyi ID. Smallpox and its eradication. Geneva: World Health Organization, 1988.
13. Eichner M. Analysis of historical data suggests long-lasting protective effects of smallpox vaccination. Am J Epidemiol 2003; 158:717–723.
14. Gani R, Leach S. Transmission potential of smallpox in contemporary populations. Nature 2001; 414:748–751.
15. Eichner M, Dietz K. Transmission potential of smallpox: estimates based on detailed data from an outbreak. Am J Epidemiol 2003; 158:110–117.

ADDITIONAL ABSTRACTS

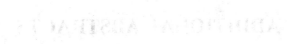

ADDITIONAL ABSTRACT

A PRIORI VERSUS A POSTERIORI RISK ASSESSMENT FOR BIOTERROR ATTACK

Eli Stern

Center for Risk Analysis, Gertner Institute, Sheba Medical Center and Tel Aviv University

Main approaches and methodologies for a priori deterministic and probabilistic risk assessment for bioterror attacks will be discussed, illustrating their major influence on emergency planning and preparedness. Definitions/descriptions, as distinct as possible, of *design basis* events (to be distinguished from *beyond design basis* events), are essential for emergency planning. Consequence modeling of the various potential bioterror events will possibly lead to their optimal classification/ranking according to severity and likelihood. One of the most crucial, rather urgent, tasks in case of a bioterror event, is not only to properly *identify* the particular bio-agent involved in the attack, but also to estimate the *size* and *severity* of the event, i.e, inter alia, the bio-agent's main modes of dispersion and hence, public exposures. Such estimations serve as vital tools for any decision-making process, concerning the optimal measures to be taken in order to minimize exposures of members of the public and the population at large to the bio-agent. The *enormous variety* of potential modes of bioterror attacks, may lead to significant gaps and differences between *real-time* and *a priori* risk assessments. Real-time risk assessment methodologies will be discussed, emphasizing the fact that they should be designed to provide experts with maximum flexibility to fit them to any particular, rather unpredictable, circumstances.

Of course, good, high level real-time risk assessments are indispensable as far as *reliable risk communication* is concerned.

IMPACT OF THE PROLIFERATION OF WEAPONS OF MASS DESTRUCTION ON THE STABILITY IN THE MIDDLE EAST

M.K. Shiyyab

Director, The cooperative Monitoring Center — Amman

The Middle East faces all kinds of security threats. One major threat is the widespread escalation of conventional military hardware and the proliferation of WMD and their delivery systems.

Greater awareness of the nature of the threat of super-terrorism since September 11 logically demands more serious consideration of the appropriate responses. Of these, the least innovation and least promising would be a familiar rehearsal of the benefits of global arms control treaties. Not only are terrorists not party to these treaties; some state leakers are also not parties to all of them; some are, but their signature is effectively worthless.

Chemical and biological materials pose a growing threat. They share with the nuclear weapons the awful potential of being used in a single attack to inflict mass casualties. While rapid growth and scientific advances in the biotechnology sector hold out the prospect of prevention and cure for many diseases, they also increase opportunities for the development of deadly new ones. That a high-damage attack has not occurred is not a cause for complacency, but a call for urgent prevention.

States parties to the Biological and Toxin Weapons Convention (BTWC) should without delay return to negotiations for a credible verification protocol, inviting the active participation of the biotechnology industry. These states must also increase bilateral diplomatic pressure to universalize membership. Furthermore, finding approaches that support, complement, and reinforce the BWC without going back to failed initiatives is a real challenge.

Biotechnology is a fast-changing field. Convergence of factors gives great cause for concern. Biotech companies are not only large pharmaceuticals, but also small units of creative, unregulated scientists, rather like in information technology (IT), brilliantly pushing the scientific frontiers, but in many cases lacking the maturity to think through consequences.

235

Terrorism attacks the values that lie at the heart of the Charter of the United Nations: respect for human rights; the rule of law; rules of war that protect civilians; tolerance among peoples and nations; and the peaceful resolution of conflict. Terrorism flourishes in environments of despair, humiliation, poverty, political oppression, extremism, and human rights abuse; it also flourishes in contexts of regional conflict and foreign occupation; and it profits from weak state capacity to maintain law and order.

In the Middle East, the best counterterrorism strategy should buy time and reduce the scale of the problem. It does not bring stability and security in the face of the broader problems in the region *unless* a political solution has been achieved. A major breakthrough in the Arab–Israeli conflict and a stable Iraq could change the rules very rapidly.

Much depends on our willingness to look at the broader causes of terrorism, discourage state terrorism and failed regimes, and avoid becoming committed to the wrong regimes and wrong causes.

The Middle East should emerge as peaceful, multinational and multicultural region where people respect each other's separate identity yet cherish their common heritage that is dominated by rationalism and sanity, free from religious and nationalistic fanaticism.

THE ROLE OF RISK ASSESSMENT IN PREPARING THE HEALTH-CARE SYSTEM FOR BIOTERRORISM AND NATURAL EPIDEMICS

Meir Oren

M.D., M.SC., M.P.H. Director General,
The Hillel-Yaffe Medical Center, Israel

Chairman, The National Committee of Hospital Preparedness
for Biological Exceptional Scenario (BW, Bioterrorism),
The Ministry of Health
oren@hy.health.gov.il

An exceptional biological incident, whether natural or an intentional act of bioterrorism, presents a challenge at the national level primarily for the health-care system, although not for it alone.

A review of the various agents, bacteria, viruses, and toxins, and the three categories classified by the American Centers for Disease Control (CDC) would suffice to denote threatening factors and possible scenarios.

A system's preparedness for coping successfully under such circumstances can be tested by its structural and process components, and by results – how well the system coped successfully, or failed to cope, with a given exceptional biological incident situation.

Successful containment is dependent on an efficient public heath-care system; a monitoring system that is *sufficiently sensitive and specific* to detect and identify exceptional morbidity *in real time or near real time*; a good primary health-care system in the community; an efficient hospitalization system with a good and flexible comprehensive hospitalization operational capability; a network of First Responders; and cooperative and organizational functions, and personnel.

The response capability of the public-health system is tested when the need arises for: an intensive epidemiological investigation on a large scale; a mass immunization project or a rapid distribution of drugs to an extensive population in a very short space of time; coordination between the various components of the health-care system, between the various components of each of the diverse agencies that interface with it, and between each of these agencies with the health-care system; development of the capability to hospitalize on a large-scale, even under conditions of isolation necessary to cope with any epidemic-generating agent; or to provide long-term mechanical respiration for a large number of patients, including children. The mix of public and private hospitalization services is critically significant when defining the hospitalization response capability at the regional and national levels, as is coping with emergency situations and preventing panic, at the national level, among the general public, as well as among public health personnel.

Preparedness and readiness for an exceptional biological incident from natural causes is a prerequisite for success in coping with an intentional incident of any kind due to bioterrorism since successful differential diagnosis between natural as opposed to nonnatural causes is very problematic, while attempts to provide different solutions for either case are not recommended for reasons of logistics and intelligence analysis.

Managing the imparting of know-how, maintaining operational alertness and readiness, *real time or near real time* monitoring of exceptional diseases, immediate intervention of public health agencies, and ensuring hospitalization surge capacity at times of crisis are all essential at the national level.

The degree of readiness during an emergency is modular and is made up of layer upon layer: readiness for an ordinary mass-injury incident, a toxicological or a chemical incident, a biological or a radiological incident, and various combinations of them all.

Successful containment is conditional on ongoing, thorough, and comprehensive implementation by the health-care system, as well as by the whole gamut of systems that interface with it, and in the successful coordination between all these bodies.

SUSCEPTIBILITY OF *B. ANTHRACIS* TO VARIOUS ANTIBACTERIAL AGENTS AND THEIR TIME–KILL ACTIVITY

Abed Athamna[1] and Ethan Rubinstein[2]
[1]*The Triangle Research and Development Center, Kfar-Qaraa, Israel and* [2]*Infectious Diseases Unit, Sheba Medical Center, Tel Aviv University School of Medicine, Tel Hashomer, Israel*

Anthrax has been the recent focus of attention as a potential biological warfare agent. It has been estimated that 50 kg of *Bacillus anthracis* spores released upwind over a population center of 500,000 would result in up to 95,000 fatalities, with an additional 123,000 persons incapacitated from inhalational anthrax.

Methods of prevention of inhalational anthrax include: protective masks capable of filtering 1–5 µm particles, appropriate sheltering, use of pre- and postexposure vaccination, and preventive and therapeutic antibiotic regimens. Recently in the United States, antibiotic prophylaxis has been administered to 32,000 individuals suspected to have been exposed to anthrax. Until the recent bioterror attack in the United States, the recommended antibiotics had not been tested in cases of human anthrax but only in a monkey model with doses of ciprofloxacin, doxycycline, and penicillin mimicking human pharmacokinetics.

The importance of antibiotic prophylaxis received special interest, mainly because of the current shortage of vaccine and lack of commercially available toxin-neutralizing agents (antitoxins).

Although the in vitro susceptibility of representative *B. anthracis* strains has been tested using a wide variety of antibiotics, little is known about the rate of bacterial killing by these agents.

It is accepted that the emergence of antibiotic resistance is a global phenomenon that is on the increase and is partially related to extensive antibiotic usage. Moreover, resistant mutants may depend on the rate of bacterial killing; the more rapid the kill rate the less likely the chance for the emergence of resistant strains. In addition, rapid killing may diminish bacterial toxin formation, and thus reduce resulting tissue damage.

In our studies [1–4] we determined the susceptibility and the rate of kill of various antibacterial agents against two nonpathogenic strains of *B. anthracis* (STi and Sterne). In addition, selection of resistant isolates was addressed too.

The results of our studies expand on the current spectrum of agents recommended for the treatment of anthrax and add several new options, such as other fluoroquinolones, amoxicillin, rifampicin, and quinupristin/dalfopristin, as potential therapeutic agents.

References

1. Athamna A, Athamna M, Nura A, Shlyakov E, Bast DJ, Farrell D, Rubinstein E. Is in vitro antibiotic combination more effective than single-drug therapy against anthrax? Antimicrob Agents Chemother 2005; 49:1323–1325.
2. Athamna A, Athamna M, Abu-Rashed N, Medlej B, Bast DJ, Rubinstein E. Selection of *Bacillus anthracis* isolates resistant to antibiotics. J Antimicrob Chemother 2004; 54:424–428.
3. Athamna A, Athamna M, Medlej B, Bast DJ, Rubinstein E. In vitro post-antibiotic effect of fluoroquinolones, macrolides, beta-lactams, tetracyclines, vancomycin, clindamycin, linezolid, chloramphenicol, quinupristin/dalfopristin and rifampicin on *Bacillus anthracis*. J Antimicrob Chemother 2004; 53:609–615.
4. Athamna A, Massalha M, Athamna M, Nura A, Medlej B, Ofek I, Bast D, Rubinstein E. In vitro susceptibility of *Bacillus anthracis* to various antibacterial agents and their time-kill activity. J Antimicrob Chemother 2004; 53:247–251.

NATURAL OR INTENTIONAL FOOD CONTAMINATION? HOW CAN WE KNOW?

Daniel Cohen
Department of Epidemiology and Preventive Medicine, Sackler Faculty of Medicine, Tel Aviv University and the Tel Aviv University Center for the Study of Bioterrorism, Tel Aviv, Israel

Salmonella and *Shigella* species, *Escherichia coli* O157:H7, *Vibrio cholerae*, *Cryptosporidium parvum*, and Noroviruses are considered by the US Centers for Disease Control as potential candidates for intentional contamination of food and water supplies. The food- and waterborne dissemination of these organisms may lead to moderate to high morbidity rates. The case fatality rates, usually low under circumstances of natural exposure, could be higher when the population is exposed to significantly higher infectious doses of these organisms in a bioterrorism scenario. Such an attack can remain uncovered and even be sustained because of the often involvement of these organisms in naturally occurring foodborne or water-borne outbreaks.

We propose to develop an algorithm to determine the likelihood that outbreaks of disease may result from intentional contamination of food. This algorithm will use descriptive, analytical, and molecular epidemiologic tools to characterize the outbreaks. High scoring will be given to unusual characteristics related to the pathogen, its mode of transmission, and the affected population, revealed by the epidemiological investigation of the outbreaks. The validity of the criteria used for differentiation can be augmented by an extensive search of the scientific literature to establish reference ranges for characteristics of naturally occurring outbreaks and laboratory studies to assess the probability that suspected food items can be potential vehicles for the epidemic transmission of specific pathogens.

BIOTERRORISM EMERGENCY RESPONSE: CURRENT CONCEPTS AND CONTROVERSIES

Eric K. Noji

Centers for Disease Control & Prevention (CDC), Washington, DC

On January 10, 2002, President Bush signed appropriations legislation providing $2.9 billion for the Department of Health and Human Services (HHS), a tenfold increase in the department's funding for bioterrorism preparedness. The funds have been used to develop comprehensive bioterrorism preparedness plans, upgrade infectious disease surveillance and investigation through the Health Alert Network (HAN), enhance the readiness of hospital systems to deal with large numbers of casualties, expand public health laboratory and communications capacities, and improve connectivity between hospitals and city, local, and state health departments to enhance disease reporting. As the lead federal agency is preparing for the threat of bioterrorism, HHS will work closely with states, local government, and the private sector to build the needed new public health infrastructure, and to accelerate research into likely bioterror diseases. As a reflection of the need for broad-based public health involvement in terrorism preparedness and planning, staff from different agencies in HHS participated in developing a strategic weapons of mass destruction (WMD) plan, including the Centers for Disease Control and Prevention (CDC), Health Resources and Services Administration (HRSA), and Office of Emergency Preparedness. The CDC will target state and local programs supporting bioterrorism, infectious diseases, and public health emergency preparedness activities state-wide. The HRSA will provide funding, which will be used by states to create regional hospital plans to respond in the event of a bioterrorism attack.

Future goals of federal public health preparedness efforts include:

- Having at least one epidemiologist in each metropolitan area with a population greater than 500,000
- Developing an education and training plan that will reach health professionals, emergency room physicians and nurses, local public

health officials, and the public with information relating to bioterrorism, new and emerging diseases, and other infectious agents
- Targeting bioterrorism research to new vaccines, antiviral drugs,
  and new diagnostic tools to better protect against biologics

This presentation outlines steps for strengthening public health and health-
care capacity to protect the population against these dangers. The health-
care industry and traditional health-care organization must join with public
health departments, law enforcement and intelligence, emergency management, and defense agencies to address potential national security threats.

PREPAREDNESS AND RESPONSE FOR BIOTERRORISM INVOLVING THE FOOD SUPPLY

Jeremy Sobel

Foodborne and Diarrheal Diseases Branch, Centers for Disease Control and Prevention, Atlanta, GA, USA

Deliberate contamination of food with biologic agents has already been perpetrated in the United States. The food supply is increasingly characterized by centralized production and processing, and wide distribution of products. The proportion of foods that are imported is steadily increasing in most countries. Thus, deliberate contamination of a food product at a single major point of production, processing, or distribution could cause an outbreak with many illnesses dispersed over wide geographic areas. Depending on the biological agent and contaminated food, such an outbreak could present variously as a slow, diffuse, and initially unremarkable increase in sporadic cases, one or more localized outbreaks, or an explosive epidemic suddenly producing a large number of illnesses. Early detection of any foodborne outbreak is critical, because the rapidity with which the contaminated food is identified, the public warned, the food removed from circulation, and appropriate medical treatment is recommended may reduce the number and severity of illnesses. In the United States, the existing public health structure at the local, state, and federal level detects and responds to well over 1,000 foodborne disease outbreaks annually, often in collaboration with foods safety regulatory authorities and state departments of agriculture. The detection and control of a bioterrorist event involving the food supply would depend to a large extent on this public health infrastructure. Preparedness for such an event, therefore, entails augmenting the traditional public health infrastructure's activities of disease surveillance, laboratory detection and diagnosis, and outbreak investigation and control, along with disaster and mass casualty response and mitigation capacity. Successful control of an outbreak of naturally occurring or deliberate foodborne disease will require timely, frank, and uniform communication messages by authorities.

RISK COMMUNICATION AND PSYCHOLOGICAL IMPACT: TECHNOLOGICAL AND OPERATIONAL METHODS OF MITIGATION

Michael J. Hopmeier

President, Unconventional Concepts, Inc., USA

Key to response to any incident is the ability to protect and defend the population from harm. However, no matter the level of investment, in either time or resources, it will never be possible to fully perform this task without enlisting the aid of the population itself. Paramount in working with a population is the ability to effectively communicate with them; without communication, we have chaos.

The purpose of this communication is primarily threefold:

1. *Educate* the population *prior* to an event so they have the knowledge, skills, and abilities to effectively respond
2. *Inform* the public during an event so they have accurate information, and the level of *noise* is decreased
3. *Direct* the public so they can apply their knowledge, skills, and abilities effectively and in a concerted manner

While there are many tried and true approaches to crisis communication, the advent of new technologies, especially over the last 5 years, is now and will in the future have enormous impact on out abilities to communicate. For decades, the major forms of communication were "static" in that they were either non-changing but portable (i.e., newspapers) or dynamic yet fixed (i.e., television). Radio, during the latter part of the 20th century became more portable, as well as dynamic, but the information content (or bandwidth) was low due to the single mode of communication, sound.

Today, with the advent of the Internet, the ubiquitous presence of cell phones, pagers, and Blackberries (or Blueberries) the ability to provide an almost unlimited quantity of data, but more importantly *information* is becoming more and more common. This is not merely an issue for the developed nations, but populations around the world.

This presentation will briefly discuss some of the key issues that have traditionally been central to the idea of crisis communication, and also discuss the added dimensions, considerations, and opportunities inherent in today's new communication technologies.